Policy issues in nursing

Policy issues in nursing

Edited by
Jane Robinson
Alastair Gray
Ruth Elkan

Open University Press
Milton Keynes · Philadelphia

Open University Press
Celtic Court
22 Ballmoor
Buckingham
MK18 1XW

and
1900 Frost Road, Suite 101
Bristol, PA 19007, USA

First Published 1992
Reprinted 1993

British Library Cataloguing-in-Publication Data

Policy issues in nursing.
  I. Robinson, Jane II. Gray, Alastair
  III. Elkan, Ruth
  610.7306

  ISBN 0-335-09467-8
  ISBN 0-335-09466-X pbk

Library of Congress Cataloging-in-Publication Data

Policy issues in nursing/Jane Robinson, Alastair Gray, Ruth Elkan,
  editors.
      p. cm.
    Includes bibliographical references and index.
    ISBN 0-335-09466-X (paperback) – ISBN 0-335-09467-8 (hardback)
    1. Nursing – Government policy – Great Britain. 2. Nursing.
  I. Robinson, Jane, 1935– . II. Gray, Alastair, 1953– .
  III. Elkan, Ruth, 1954– .
    [DNLM: 1. Nursing – trends – Great Britain. WY 300 FA1 P76]
  RT11.P65   1991
  362.1'73'0941 – dc20
  DNLM/DLC
  for Library of Congress   91-24012
                                                          CIP

Typeset by Rowland Phototypesetting Limited
Bury St Edmunds, Suffolk
Printed in Great Britain by
Biddles Ltd, Guildford and King's Lynn

Contents

List of contributors

Jim Buchan is a Research Fellow at the Institute of Manpower Studies, where he specializes in researching issues relating to the recruitment, retention and remuneration of health service professionals. He is currently working as a visiting Fellow at the King's Fund Institute. From 1984 to 1987 he worked for the Royal College of Nursing.

Ruth Elkan is a sociologist with research interests in the health and social services labour force. She has studied trade unionism, residential provision in the community and nurse education policy research. She is currently research associate at the Department of Nursing Studies, University of Nottingham, researching into Project 2000.

Alastair Gray is an economist with research interests in several aspects of health and health care, especially concerning the health service labour force and nurses in particular. He has previously worked at the University of Aberdeen and the Open University, and is currently based at the Centre for Socio-Legal Studies, Wolfson College, Oxford.

Nicky James is a nurse and sociologist, graduating from the University of Aberdeen. She worked in the voluntary sector as co-ordinator of the Homeless Alcoholics Recovery Project and then in the Birmingham Law Courts setting up a Court Alcohol Service. She has a long-term research interest in hospices and nurses' contributions to health. She is senior lecturer in the Department of Nursing Studies at the University of Nottingham and is working with the University Hospital neonatal nursing service researching workload.

Dirk Keyzer is a general and orthopaedic trained nurse and has studied nursing at Manchester University and London University Institute of Education. He has a specific research interest in the distribution of power and control in nursing organizations and its impact on the development of a practitioner role for the registered nurse. He is currently Professor in the Department of Community Health at Deakin University, Geelong, Victoria, Australia.

Leila Lessof qualified in medicine and undertook postgraduate training to become a consultant Radiologist. Whilst working as a consultant she became increasingly interested in broader issues relating to health and health services and retrained in public health medicine becoming a District Medical Officer to Islington Health Authority in 1982. In 1990 she became Director of Public Health to Parkside Health Authority.

Martin McKee qualified in medicine at the Queen's University of Belfast. He is a senior lecturer in the Department of Public Health and Policy at the London School of Hygiene and Tropical Medicine, where he is responsible for co-ordinating the Department's European public health activities. His doctoral thesis was on the out of hours work of junior doctors.

Anne Marie Rafferty is a graduate nurse from the University of Edinburgh and is completing a doctorate in the history of nurse education policy at Oxford University. She was affiliated to the Wellcome Unit for the History of Medicine in Oxford before taking up a lectureship in the Nursing Studies Department at the University of Nottingham. She has undertaken clinical research into postoperative backache and is currently researching leadership development in nursing.

Jane Robinson is professor and head of the Department of Nursing Studies at the University of Nottingham. She is an orthopaedic and general trained nurse, a health visitor and health visitor tutor. Her research interests lie in health service evaluation, especially concerning the ways in which policy-makers define and monitor the roles of subordinate occupational groups. Prior to moving to Nottingham she was director of the Nursing Policy Studies Centre at the University of Warwick where she collaborated with (amongst others) Alastair Gray, Ruth Elkan and John Stilwell on studies of various aspects of the nursing labour force.

Kate Robinson is a registered general nurse and health visitor, and holds degrees in history and health studies. Her research work has largely been focused on community nursing, although she has more general interests in nursing as work and the nursing workforce. She works as a teacher of health workers, and is particularly interested in promoting open learning and creating accessible routes into education. She is currently Dean of the Faculty of Health Care and Social Studies at Luton College of Higher Education.

Jane Salvage trained as a general nurse after completing a degree in English Literature. Her interest in and experience of the politics of nursing led her to study for an MSc in the sociology of health and illness. She has also written and lectured on a range of nursing issues. At the beginning of 1991 she was appointed to the post of regional officer for nursing, midwifery and social work in the World Health Organization's European Regional Office in Copenhagen. Her former post, as director of the Nursing Developments Programme, King's Fund Centre for Health Services Development, enabled her to explore new ways of empowering nurses to improve their practice and to value themselves more highly.

John Stilwell is director of the Health Services Research Unit at the University of Warwick. After studying Politics, Philosophy and Economics at Jesus College Oxford he worked as an economist at Essex and Strathclyde Universities before specializing in health economics at the Department of Social Medicine, University of Birmingham.

Chris West has been the District General Manager of the Portsmouth and South East Hampshire Health Authority since 1984. He holds an MSc in Business Administration from Durham University and is a member of the Audit Commission.

Preface

Some feminist writers have argued that in a world which no longer discriminated against women, nursing would be far more highly rewarded. But is this true? Was nursing undervalued because it was done by women or were women simply allocated to the less remunerative tasks? The latter is a simpler and more plausible explanation, for there is a crucial distinction to be made between the usefulness of something and what people would actually pay to get hold of it. Price is determined, not just by need but by the ease with which others can supply it. Nursing was a bit like water; fundamental to life but has, for the most part, in the past been readily available. These, at least, are the arguments which have held true until now. Their rationale is beginning to be challenged, however, in the light of ... demographic, social and economic forces.... Paradoxically, as more women enter the labour market, the supply of cheap female labour to nursing is beginning (because of greater alternative employment opportunities) to diminish. In addition, women are beginning successfully to demand remuneration on the basis of equal pay for equal work.

(Strong and Robinson 1988: 48)

The idea for an edited collection on policy issues in nursing came about when the Nursing Policy Studies Centre (NPSC) at the University of Warwick was being wound down in 1989 after a short but productive existence of just under five years. During those preceding five years the Centre's research has focused on aspects of some of the most fundamental changes which had taken place within the NHS during the second half of the 1980s and through this we had been in touch with a broad range of opinions and ideas on health care and on nursing.

Justice has probably been done to the broad picture of change which we analysed following our four-year study of the introduction of general management into the NHS through the recording of our findings and interpretations in *The NHS Under New Management* (Strong and Robinson 1990), but there was still much about nursing which had not been captured in our reports. Two predominant but often conflicting approaches had emerged from the observations made of nursing during the Centre's four and a half year history. First, some nurses around the country were trying to change the organization of nursing work in terms both of the quality of care they provided for the patient and for their own sense of meaning and job satisfaction. Their approach was broadly holistic and was underpinned by ethical considerations. They argued strongly that clinically based nurses should have control of the assessment, planning, delivery and evaluation of individualized nursing care, and they advocated appropriate, broad educational preparation for the job. The second approach to the organization of nursing work was rooted in a rational–scientific framework which placed nursing within the context of labour supply and demand. Education here was much more about acquiring the necessary competence to carry out health care tasks within the most cost-efficient division of labour. We observed also the way in which those working within the first approach often felt it necessary to justify their position in terms of the second, arguing, for example, that the organization of nursing care which they advocated would result in a more cost effective deployment of the nursing workforce with better retention of qualified nursing staff. Although touching on some of the ramifications of these two approaches in its research, the Centre had not attempted to explore them in any depth. It was with these omissions in mind that the editors, Alastair Gray (who carried out for the Centre the first global nursing economics literature review, Gray 1987), Ruth Elkan and Jane Robinson approached the contributors to this edited collection – for we knew of them as people with strong views about nursing, and the direction it could, or should, take. Our brief to them was minimal: to describe from their own perspective (whether that consisted of an academic or practical viewpoint) their ideas on past, current or future policies for nursing. We chose contributors quite deliberately from a mixture of nurses and non-nurses. Hence, amongst the latter there is a district general manager (Chris West), a health economist (John Stilwell), two community physicians (Leila Lessof and Martin McKee) and an operational researcher (Jim Buchan). The nurses comprise the new regional officer for nursing, midwifery and social work in the World Health Organization's European Region who was formerly the director of nursing developments at the King Edward's Hospital Fund for London (Jane Salvage), three nurse academics and teachers (Nicky James, Anne Marie Rafferty and Kate Robinson), and a nurse civil servant (Dirk Keyzer). We believed that, by leaving them to set their own agenda, there was a strong probability that at least some of the tensions and pressures which currently underpin many of the debates about nursing and its future would emerge. We were not disappointed. Different contributors have selected different aspects of nursing for consideration and more divergent than convergent ideas emerge about how nurses' roles could, or should, be structured and managed. All of the ideas raise interesting questions for debate.

The introduction to this book raises many of the themes and issues which emerge in subsequent chapters. The introductory chapter describes the setting up of the NPSC at Warwick University as a case study in the establishment of a tradition of critical nursing policy research. The chapter then looks at how the Centre used its first major piece of research into the implementation of the Griffiths reforms in the NHS (Strong and Robinson 1988) as a vehicle for carrying out nursing policy research. The question 'what is nursing policy?' is raised in this introduction. Most of the subsequent chapters also deal with this question, either explicitly or implicitly, and the range of interpretations of 'nursing policy' is very great. Elements of the two predominant approaches to nursing policy issues outlined above are evident in most of the contributory chapters. While Jane Salvage's chapter (1), with its emphasis on the ideology and content of the 'new' professional nursing, best exemplifies an analysis of the first approach, John Stilwell's and Jim Buchan's chapters (7 and 3), with their emphases respectively on cost efficiency in the deployment of nursing labour, and nurse workforce planning, best exemplify the second.

The question of who determines nursing policy is raised by several contributors. The introductory chapter draws attention to the way in which nurses are rarely involved in policy-making but instead, simply acquiesce to others' formulations of nursing issues. Anne Marie Rafferty takes up this theme (Chapter 6), exploring, through an historical perspective, nursing's virtual absence from policy-making arenas. Chris West, too, charts the peaks and troughs in nursing's influence on public policy during the past 40 years (Chapter 4). And finally, Martin McKee and Leila Lesoff (Chapter 5), who look at the way in which doctors and government have played a substantial part in defining the extended role of the nurse, also illustrate how nurses may be drawn into accepting others' formulations of their 'proper' role.

The professionalization of nursing is also a subject to which several contributors make reference. Jane Salvage, Kate Robinson, Dirk Keyzer (Chapter 9), Chris West and Anne Marie Rafferty all make clear that although the professionalization of nursing is rarely an explicitly articulated policy objective, it nevertheless forms an important hidden agenda behind many of the reforms and policies advocated by nurses.

Finally, almost all the contributors place nursing within a wider framework of women's work. Jim Buchan and Drs McKee and Lessof point to the changing position of women in the labour market and their heightened aspirations, indicating that employers will need to develop new and creative ways of recruiting, retaining and motivating the nursing workforce. By contrast Kate Robinson's concern (Chapter 2) is with gender and race in determining subordinate positions both within the NHS and in the wider society. Nicky James's interest (Chapter 8) lies in the relationship between the ideology of women's caring role within the family and women's caring role within the nursing workforce.

The emergence of these diverse ideas is important as, for reasons of demography, potential labour shortages, feminist theory or even the challenges raised by questioning nurses themselves, nursing is, after a period of relative obscurity, once again visible on the public policy agenda. Yet, in the absence of a clearly defined power base or any apparent consensus over the strategic direction which nursing should take, the occupation is still vulnerable to the passing fashions of successive health policy-makers. For, as the introductory chapter makes clear, a crucial finding which emerged from the Nursing Policy Studies Centre's work was nursing's lack of importance as a matter of serious policy concern. Nurses appear to have been completely powerless to influence the systematic dismantling of their own control of the management of nursing and its budgets as the implementation of the Griffiths Report (DHSS 1983) throughout the second half of the 1980s showed. At the time of writing it is the future of the statutory bodies and the funding and regulation of nurse education that are under major review. Unless nurses set all contemporary change within the broader context of what is happening in health care they are likely to react parochially and with the introspection which has characterized so many of nursing's responses in the past. However, if there is a new commitment on the part of governments to take nursing issues seriously in the final years of the twentieth century, then there is every reason to acknowledge that nurses wish to be party to the decisions which shape their future, and to make explicit some of nursing's fundamental concerns.

Jane Robinson

Acknowledgements

The editors extend their thanks to all the contributors to this book. Without their hard work, enthusiasm and willingness to meet deadlines this book would not have been possible.

Thanks are also extended to the members of staff in the Department of Nursing Studies, University of Nottingham, for their tolerance of the inevitable preoccupation which accompanies the editing of a book. We thank especially Liz LeQuelenec for her invaluable assistance with the preparation of the final manuscript.

We also acknowledge with thanks the pioneering work of Dr Rosemary White who negotiated with the King Edward's Hospital Fund for London the original funding for the establishment of the Nursing Policy Studies Centre at the University of Warwick. Despite its relatively short lifespan, the Centre's existence from 1985 to 1988 enabled us to establish a critical policy analysis approach to nursing issues. This book attempts to foster and to continue this tradition.

List of abbreviations

AHA	Area Health Authority
AIDS	Acquired Immune Deficiency Syndrome
AMA	American Medical Association
BMA	British Medical Association
BTEC	Business and Technical Education Council
CHSC	Central Health Services Council
CHSR	Centre for Health and Social Research
CMO	Chief Medical Officer
CNO	Chief Nursing Officer
COHSE	Confederation of Health Service Employees
DHA	District Health Authority
DHSS	Department of Health and Social Security
DoE	Department of Employment
DoH	Department of Health
EMS	Emergency Medical Services
EN	Enrolled Nurse
ENB	English National Board
GNC	General Nursing Council
HIV	Human Immunodeficiency Virus
HMC	Hospital Management Committee
IMS	Institute of Manpower Studies
JBCNS	Joint Board of Clinical Nursing Studies
MLNS	Ministry of Labour and National Service
MoH	Ministry of Health

NALGO   National Association of Local Government Officers
NAO   National Audit Office
NCVQ   National Council for Vocational Qualifications
NHS   National Health Service
NHSTA   National Health Service Training Authority
NO   Nursing Officer
NPSC   Nursing Policy Studies Centre
NUPE   National Union of Public Employees
ONDU   Oxford Nursing Development Unit
OPEC   Organization of Petroleum Exporting Countries
OTA   Occupational Therapist Aide
RAWP   Resource Allocation Working Party
RCN   Royal College of Nursing
RHA   Regional Health Authority
RHB   Regional Hospital Board
RNO   Regional Nursing Officer
SAC   Standing Advisory Committee
SHHD   Scottish Home and Health Department
SNAC   Standing Nursing Advisory Committee
TUC   Trades Union Congress
TVEI   Technical and Vocational Education Initiative
UKCC   United Kingdom Central Council for Nursing, Midwifery
          and Health Visiting
WHO   World Health Organization
WO   Welsh Office
wte   whole time equivalent
YTS   Youth Training Scheme

Introduction: Beginning the study of nursing policy

Jane Robinson

January 1985 was a time when nursing's importance as a matter of public policy concern was apparently at its lowest ebb. The early implementation of the Griffiths Report (DHSS 1983, 1984), with the introduction of general management into the NHS, was already having an impact. Reports were emerging informally, and in the nursing press, of chief nursing officers at district and regional levels of the health service losing in some instances their jobs; in many cases their control over the nursing budget; and in others, their line management of nursing. In the spring of 1986 the Royal College of Nursing (RCN) launched a major campaign in the national press in order to draw the public's attention to these perceived injustices. The purchase of a full page spread in the *Sunday Times* to ask wittily whether 'the general manager knows his coccyx from his humerus?' certainly put the RCN into a new light in terms of its ability to use the media. However, at major and probably unacceptable financial cost, the campaign proved to be almost completely unsuccessful in stemming the tide of these changes in the management of the nursing labour force.

It was ironic, therefore, that at the same time as these events were taking place, the Nursing Policy Studies Centre (NPSC) at Warwick University (funded by the King Edward's Hospital Fund for London – an institution that was itself deeply committed to the reform of the NHS) should not only have been established, but also given the freedom to choose its own research topic within its overall funding framework. The Centre had a constitution with three major objectives:

1 To develop the theoretical evaluation of nursing policy.

2 To influence the making of policy so that nurses could make the optimal contribution to health service and health care policy in all sectors and at all levels of the health care system.
3 To involve nurses and to create greater awareness amongst nurses and others of nursing policy issues (NPSC 1988).

The initial construction of a programme designed to meet these objectives demanded prior attention to several underlying issues. Firstly what did the term *nursing policy* mean, and what was the justification for sub-dividing a broad academic area such as policy studies in order to concentrate on one, albeit large, section of the health care labour force? Emerging as the Centre's director from the relative obscurity of health policy research, I found the whole notion of nursing policy studies tantalizing. There was no such thing as *medical* policy studies. Why then should nursing need such specialized attention? The nursing lobby which had supported the Centre's establishment probably saw the Centre simply as completing the triumvirate of nursing research centres in England, the other two (for nursing practice and education) having been created during the 1970s. The august members of the Centre's Advisory Board gave the impression that the nature of nursing policy is self-evident and certainly did not appear to share my scepticism about the undertaking on which we had embarked. At one of the Board's early meetings it was suggested that nursing policy studies is simply about studying the kinds of matters dealt with by the Salmon Report:

> In top management nurses formulate nursing policy and organise its implementation by others, whose functions they coordinate. The primary objects of nursing policy are a high quality nursing care for the patients and the training of nurses in accordance with professional requirements. A principal administrative function is reconciling the two objects in a practical plan. The personnel function is equally important, for the whole tone of a hospital and the happiness of the patients and the people who work in it are deeply influenced by the nursing heads.
>
> (Ministry of Health, Scottish Home and
> Health Department 1966: 57)

In the light of what was currently happening to nursing this conceptualization of the tasks in hand hardly appeared credible. It seemed that any serious work on policies in relation to nursing would require the suspension of judgement over many currently held assumptions about the nature of the occupation. From earlier studies on child abuse (Robinson 1979), health visiting (Robinson 1982), and perinatal mortality (Robinson 1989) I was fascinated by the persuasive notion of consensus which is conveyed in so many policy texts. It appeared that some members of the Centre's Advisory Board were unable to recognize the conflict of interests at play when certain policies are defeated and successful ones are then presented as the consensus view; although nursing in general has had a long history of losing out to more powerful interests.

Seizing the initiative and determining the course of events in policy matters appears to be crucially dependent on the holding of power: power not only to ensure that an issue reaches – or fails to reach – the public agenda, but power also to define the issue in such a way as to bring about particular ends. Nursing after Griffiths had lost any illusion of the power it might once have possessed and our task of unpacking the notion of nursing policy was clearly going to require that we undertake an area of empirical research where the occupation could be studied against the backdrop of other vested interests.

Second, the Centre's resources were relatively slender and nursing is a vast occupation containing within it numerous sub-groups. Concentration on policy issues of general concern to nurses appeared to be a major requisite. The reason that the management of the nursing labour force following the implementation of the Griffiths Inquiry Report was chosen as the Centre's initial area of study lay in the opportunity it gave to research an issue of immediate relevance to nurses across all the clinical specialisms as well as addressing some of the crucial policy questions which had never been considered before in relation to nursing.

The strategy appeared to pay off. Although core financial support for the Centre was never achieved beyond the pump-priming provided by the King Edward's Hospital for London, the four and a half years of the Centre's existence proved to be highly productive. The 'Griffiths research' (as it became known) resulted in three reports (Robinson and Strong 1987; Strong and Robinson 1988; Robinson *et al.* 1989a) and one book (Strong and Robinson 1990). The Centre's research also resulted in three further reports on commissioned research (Gray 1987; Robinson and Elkan 1989; Robinson *et al.* 1989b); this edited collection; and several papers which reflected on the lessons to which the experience gave rise. As a result a critical policy analysis approach to nursing issues has been established.

Critical policy analysis

Of what does this critical policy analysis consist? It is an approach to policy issues rooted in reflexivity and in the constant attempt to suspend judgement over the prevailing explanations of how policy comes about. Several analysts have set out both the theoretical and practical approaches to critical policy analysis. Rein (1983) asserts its method is 'value critical' for it probes the value assumptions which organize the evidence. He urges the importance of a sceptical approach to policy issues and challenges the analyst to question her own values as well as those she seeks to study. He distinguishes between the 'value critical' approach where 'seeing is believing' and the 'value committed' approach where 'believing is seeing'. Rein argues that each has its place in policy analysis but that the value critical approach is essential where deeply held values are challenged.

This stance was crucially important in the Griffiths research where ethnographic research methods appeared to be the only way to begin to understand and to explain the complex phenomena we sought to study and where, inevitably, as a nurse, I saw the world through 'nursing eyes'. Reflecting on the NHS through participant observation needed an 'outsider' to help to interpret what I, the 'insider', was observing. This was achieved by my co-researcher at that time, Philip Strong, who not only was not a nurse but was a sociologist, a man and (crucially) admitted to knowing nothing about nursing when he began the work. His reflection acted as a foil to mine as we sought to make sense of the various observations we each made and of the stories we were told by the different respondents in our fieldwork.

The empirical study: methods

In Year One we carried out detailed exploratory work and on the basis of this preliminary research decided to focus on the district tier of management. Seven widely varying districts were selected for particular study, three of them with a national reputation for innovation in the management of nursing (although data were gathered from a good many other districts). These districts were studied in two rounds of research. The first started in January 1986 and lasted six months. In this period, most of the senior managers then in post were interviewed. The second, much more rapid round, came a year later in 1987 when just the district general managers and chief nurse advisers were spoken to. But if district was the core, it was not the whole of our study: DHSS, regions, units and professional gatherings also came in for some share of our research. The final part of the study comprised a questionnaire survey of 200 chief nurse advisers carried out during its fourth year in 1988 and to which an 81 per cent response rate was achieved. All of these findings, plus the observations made during the Centre's commissioned work and on the work of other authors, came to inform what has become the ongoing analysis of policy related to nursing.

The empirical study: initial findings

What were the key findings from the empirical research? First, that many of our respondents (including nurses) were enthusiastic about the need for managerial reform of the NHS. This may have been the first flush of enthusiasm and most of those interviewed had done rather well as a result of Griffiths. Nevertheless there was a widespread feeling that change of this order was inevitable.

Second, and crucially, was nursing's invisibility to virtually everyone except nurses. Our 'mulling over' of the meaning of our observations crystallized one day in that flash of insight which characterizes the research enterprise and which we immediately labelled 'The Black Hole Theory of Nursing'. In general, it appeared that I had been observing nurses, many (but not all) of whom seemed defensively unable to see their work within a broad policy context. Philip Strong, on the other hand, had observed general managers and doctors who displayed the most profound ignorance about pressing nursing issues and practice. It appeared that even where nurses had become nationally known within nursing for taking their work forward in creative and imaginative ways, the local general managers and doctors apparently could remain profoundly ignorant of such innovations. We suddenly realized that despite the impressive statistics (half a million workforce in the UK) nursing is relatively unimportant to government and to managers in comparison with medicine. It was *medicine* that the Griffiths reforms sought to control – *nursing* was merely caught in the crossfire! The tensions to which this situation gave rise – the nursing group locked into the gravitational force of its internal preoccupations, and the others, on the outside, unable or unwilling to look in and comprehend the nature of nursing's dilemmas – seemed to us to be the social equivalent of an astronomical Black Hole.

One or two exceptions to this general observation did shine like beacons in a gloomy landscape. Amongst the three districts noted for their innovation in nursing management we found examples where there had been conscious planning of the support needed to provide high quality nursing advice coupled with definite strategies to recruit high calibre, highly educated nurses (although the innovations were sometimes the isolated product of nurses' initiatives unsupported by others). We also discovered that a similar but more focused commitment to innovation in nurse education was held by the most highly qualified nurses responding to our survey. We were led to the conclusion that the historic lack of critical, well-educated nurses may have accounted, in part, for nursing's inability to escape from the Black Hole. On the basis of our empirical evidence we surmised that education is a crucial factor in producing more self-confident nurses who are not afraid to take their seat at the various policy-making top tables and to make a creative contribution to the planning, delivery and evaluation of health care.

The third key finding was that nurses were the members of staff who most often raised questions of equity and humanity in health care. Financial matters preoccupied most of the managers and the district health authority meetings we observed. We saw little evidence of health authorities planning care within an overall philosophy such as Health for All or Primary Health Care. Financial fire-fighting was the order of the day.

Methodological issues

Reflexivity – the methodological stance that underpinned the Centre's approach to the entire nursing policy analysis enterprise – is characterized above all by its recognition that we are part of the social world we aim to study. Reflexivity accepts as an existential fact that there is no way that we can escape the social world. Here it differs profoundly on the one hand from positivism, with its concern with a scientific method modelled on the natural sciences and its emphasis on the hypothetico-deductive testing of theories, and on the other hand from naturalism's proposition that the social world should be studied in its 'natural' state, undisturbed by the researcher. In all of the Centre's research we accepted that we could not avoid having an effect on the social phenomena we studied. We approached our subjects, not as sources of data, but as experts with whom we ourselves had a most unusual relationship. In the Griffiths research, we were not academic ethnographers studying some strange tribe but were, in our respective ways, part of the very culture we aimed to study. Philip Strong initially may have known little about nursing, but he knew a great deal about the NHS, medicine and management. Like some of our respondents, I too had once been a nurse manager and had had a lengthy career in the NHS. We had both studied many aspects of health service organization, both held strong views about it; and both could quite well have been doing some of the jobs we were trying to study. Hence many of our interviews became a dialogue – a shared attempt to understand and to grapple with the complexities of nursing and the NHS and the tremendous changes that both were undergoing. A guiding principle of the research was that there is:

> . . . as little justification for rejecting all common-sense knowledge out of hand as there is for treating it as all 'valid in its own terms': we have no external, absolutely conclusive standard by which we judge it. Rather, we must work with what knowledge we have. . . . Similarly, instead of treating reactivity merely as a source of bias, we can exploit it. How people respond to the presence of the researcher may be as informative as how they react to other situations.
>
> (Hammersley and Atkinson 1983: 15)

Research carried out in this context undoubtedly raises the question: how does this activity differ from journalism, literature or indeed normal social intercourse? Many of the respondents we studied *were* theorists for they were trained at least in part, in social science and management theory. For our part, we saw our dialogue with them as a continual process of generating propositions and testing out explanations, trying to see if 'the fit' was right and then moving on. As a result there was a certain *disadvantage* to the different orientations which Philip Strong and I brought to the research for its original focus shifted, at least in the short term, to a study of the NHS rather than primarily of the management of nursing within it. In retrospect, this now appears to have been important for it represents another manifestation of nursing's invisibility. It did ensure, nevertheless, that my undivided attention was not turned to nursing's obscurity in policy terms until the Centre's short life span was almost complete. If the Black Hole Theory of Nursing gave us an initial, *theorizing* idea which served to describe the tensions which hold nursing in its place it was, at that stage, a different matter to begin to explain them. Indeed, we held many inconclusive discussions on the nature of the mechanisms which give rise to this state of affairs. Philip Strong saw the problem simply in terms of scarcity or a 'water and diamonds' analogy – nursing skills are plentiful, like water; brain surgeons are scarce, like diamonds. The Griffiths research did not resolve the dilemma and we continued to try to address the issue in the subsequent work from the Centre. This needed consideration of questions of gender and power. Unfortunately, we are so 'locked in' to our prior socialization and traditional ways of looking at the world that it is extraordinarily difficult to think one's way into alternative paradigms. This process constitutes the ongoing theoretical endeavour which we all share as part of re-thinking our place in the order of things and which is central to a critical policy approach to issues.

Subsequent reflection on the issues

In developing an analysis of the phenomenon of which nurses are a part it appears crucial to enquire why nursing is perceived to be so unimportant in policy terms. Why did it prove to be so easy to sweep many nurse managers aside in the reorganization following the Griffiths Report? Why is the voice of nursing still disregarded in the context of current changes to the NHS (despite nurses' very real knowledge and concern about their likely impact on some of the most disadvantaged NHS clients)? Two papers set an agenda whereby we might begin to make sense of these issues (Robinson 1990, 1991). The first concerns nursing as a women's issue, the second nursing within the context of power, politics and policy analysis. There are no definite conclusions and certainly no grand theory – perhaps grand theory should not be the aim but instead the continual process of reflection and re-interpretation. There is now, however, a fairly substantial groundswell of self-questioning by nurses which revolves around some of the following issues:

1 Nurses are virtually never involved in concrete policy decision-making processes; what may pass as a nursing decision is in reality acquiescence to others' prior formulations.
2 Issues that primarily concern nurses (for example, maintaining adequate staffing levels in order to ensure humane and equitable standards of care) are either kept off the formal policy agenda or disguised as nurses' inability to manage scarce resources adequately.
3 Contemporary health policy initiatives seek to control the apparently limitless power of medicine to expand by bringing in cost-containment policies which set nurse against nurse. The ways in which this process takes place are now well described in the North American literature (Robinson 1991; White 1985, 1986a, 1988) and they are becoming a matter for increasing concern

in the UK. Whilst for some nurses cost-containment measures provide an opportunity for enhancing their professional power and status, for others, the result is increased workload and an impoverishment of both their working conditions and their ability to deliver high standards of nursing care. For yet others, such policies jeopardize their very jobs. The 'order to care in a society that refuses to value caring' (Reverby 1987) results in conflicts which extend across the qualified/unqualified, waged/unwaged female caring divides. Other chapters in this book pick up on these tensions, for example, Kate Robinson's and Nicky James' chapters, 2 and 8, respectively, as a contrast to the positions taken by Chris West and John Stilwell later in this book, chapters 4 and 7 respectively.

4 The Black Hole of Nursing is maintained by the force of the tensions generated between these conflicting positions.

The competing groups within nursing fail to set the occupational issues within the wider socio-economic context of health care and to perceive that it is primarily through its internal divisions that nursing's subordination is maintained. Finding a common voice in nursing will only be achieved by nurses adopting a reflective stance which demands a critical evaluation of values just as much in day to day practice as in the qualitative research enterprise. Certainly we came to believe that nursing's role models lie in those highly educated nurses whom we observed taking their seat at the policy-making top tables and asserting their right to be heard, not just for nursing but across the whole spectrum of health care issues.

I

The New Nursing: Empowering patients or empowering nurses?

Jane Salvage

In this chapter Jane Salvage explores the central elements of a new professional reform movement, the 'New Nursing'. Basing her study on personal observation and a review of the nursing and sociological literature, Jane Salvage combines many of the insights of medical sociology (in particular its work on professionalism, occupational strategies and the doctor–patient relationship) with a committed yet critical nursing perspective. The result is an original and powerful critique of the New Nursing.

Introduction

British nursing has entered a period of major change, prompted by a combination of forces – including pressures from within, difficulty in recruiting and retaining staff, significant educational reform, and demands for higher status for women's work. Since the early 1980s there has been an unprecedented burst of activity leading to a variety of initiatives to reform different aspects of nursing. These emanate from many organizations and individual nurses, adopt different approaches, and advocate a wide range of solutions; they encompass scrutiny of the practice of nursing as well as of its training, structure, rewards and power. They contain broad agreement on many key issues and indeed add up to a 'movement', described in this chapter and elsewhere as 'the New Nursing'.

The theoretical perspective brought to bear on the New Nursing in this chapter is that of a nurse looking at sociology. As a clinical nurse and subsequently a journalist and commentator on nursing, I have been dismayed by the virtual absence of some key issues from debates on nursing at all levels (from practitioners to policy-makers). Although there is a long-running preoccupation with power and the control of nursing work, usually expressed as a desire for professional status, there has been a marked lack of discussion of its major themes: how the practice of nursing is shaped by social formations, the meaning of nursing work, the division of labour in health care and in nursing, and the links between nursing and women's work.

These issues are at long last beginning to be more widely discussed, within and outside nursing. My own search for insight and my interest in the politics of nursing led me to sociology, especially its health-care-related work on professionalism and occupational strategies, and on the doctor–patient relationship. It also led me to feminist theory, since it is impossible to understand nursing without acknowledging its position as a female occupation doing archetypal 'women's work'. Both disciplines contributed to my exploration of the New Nursing, and in particular of nurse–patient relationships, the cornerstone of the reform movement's ideology.

Sociological study of nursing practice is bound to encounter the tension between how care is prescribed in textbooks and courses, and how it is delivered. This is commonly described by nurses as the 'theory–practice gap', though it might more profitably be addressed in terms of a tension between the forces which shape nursing practice (internal and external) and the efforts of some nurses (including the New Nurses) to set their own agendas. Analysis of this tension places the debate in an inescapably political context: proponents of the New Nursing, building on a particular value-system, seek to widen its sphere of influence by transforming power relations.

The study that forms the core of this chapter was conducted in 1988 for an MSc course in sociology with special reference to medicine (Royal Holloway and Bedford New College, University of London). I began with a review of some current nursing literature, especially work emanating from the Oxford Nursing Development Unit (ONDU).[1] I spent a brief period in the Unit itself, and analysed three other studies of its work. Finally I explored some sociological studies of nurse–patient relationships and nurses' views of nursing. I concluded that major changes are needed in nurses' occupational socialization and the organization of hospital work if they are to practise in the way advocated; that the question 'Why now?' seeks further exploration; and that these issues are skated over in the debate within nursing (Salvage 1990a). I also contended that tough questions need to be asked about the proponents of the New Nursing; we cannot assume that they are exclusively concerned with improving patient care. The movement should also be understood as a specific occupational strategy which claims higher status for nurses (or some of them) by utilizing notions of authority (resting on positivistic science), expertise (based on good education) and responsiveness to social needs. Is this simply old-style professionalism revamped by a new élite in pursuit of their own power, or a creative attempt to seek empowerment for nurses and patients, or a bit of both?

Before discussing my study in more detail I should declare my bias. I am not only an observer of the New Nursing, but an active participant in it. The programme I direct at the King's Fund Centre for Health Services Development owes much, in its philosophy and its practice, to the nurses whose work I have analysed, not least those from the ONDU. Critique can seem more like betrayal when you are part of a movement, you share many of its ideals and its proponents are your colleagues and friends. Similarly, reminders of painful realities are sometimes misconstrued as negative attempts to hinder progress. However, the stake I have in the New Nursing makes me all the more determined to explore it critically (and to understand why I am personally attracted to it). Individual and collective self-awareness is a positive development in contemporary nursing, and I hope this chapter makes a contribution to it.

A new philosophy of nursing

The New Nursing began in the UK in the early 1970s, with the new departments of nursing in universities and polytechnics generating interest in nursing theory. They drew heavily on work from the USA, which sought to redefine the nurse's role in order to assert its unique contribution to healing (Henderson 1966), leading to claims for greater status, while the women's movement began to challenge assumptions about nursing's subordination to medicine. Meanwhile better standards of education, higher expectations and nascent consumerism provoked a reappraisal of the client/expert relationship on both sides of the Atlantic.

Key elements can be crystallized from the activities and discussions prompted by these trends. Typically today they may be identified in publications by 'academic' nurses (e.g. Chapman 1985), but also those by practitioners who have undergone higher education, such as Pearson (1983, 1988) and Wright (1986), well-known clinical leaders and exponents of the New Nursing. The distinction between nursing academics and practitioners is not clearcut.

In these publications, the key to the New Nursing is held to be its clinical base. The bureaucratic occupational model must be replaced by a professional one, with the practitioner as its linchpin; preparation for this demanding role is to be achieved via improved education. This 'new animal' (UKCC 1986a) should have greater autonomy at the centre of a new division of labour; no longer should a position of seniority mean leaving direct patient care.

Discharging the 'unique function' of the nurse (Henderson 1966, cited in virtually every text) is said to involve a systematic problem-solving approach and scientifically derived knowledge. It also requires different relationships with patients – moving away from the biomedical model, which views medical intervention as the solution to health problems, towards a holistic approach enabling the patient's active participation in care. The patient is seen as a whole person for whom all aspects of healing work are crucial, including 'basic nursing care' such as bathing and toiletting. These tasks must therefore be restored to a central place in the work of the qualified nurse, since they are just as important as the supposedly more skilled, 'scientific' tasks handed down to nurses from doctors. As Armstrong notes, the form and nature of the portrayal of the nurse–patient relationship underwent 'a fundamental reformulation' in nursing textbooks from the early 1970s (Armstrong 1983a: 457). The nurse's caring role should no longer be restricted to biological functions, but should acknowledge the subjectivity of nurse and patient in a two-way relationship.

The nursing philosophy summarized above, despite its sometimes pejorative association with a 'remote, professionalising élite' (e.g. Melia 1987: 158), has been used as a framework for practice, notably in centres of excellence such as nursing development units. It is also apparent in innovations such as the nurse practitioner role in primary healthcare (DHSS 1986a). Its influence over the Project 2000 education proposals is marked (UKCC 1986a). Finally the staff organizations, notably the Royal College of Nursing, play a key part in developing, disseminating and reproducing it (e.g. in Clay 1987).

My study focused on the idea of 'partnership' between nurses and patients as a key aspect to the New Nursing. It is a concept that raises questions about the links between the rhetoric of ideology and daily experience; highlights the relationship between expert and client; and touches on 'consumerism'. After exploring the notion of partnership as ideology, I look at partnership in practice, and the implications for nursing. The study is based on readings in the sociology and nursing literature; personal experience as a nurse; and observation of nursing as a development worker and as a sociologist.

The ideology of partnership

What is the theory of partnership? Project 2000 (UKCC 1986a) proposes 'new concepts underpinning education and practice' in nursing. These include enhancing the patient's health knowledge and skills; maximum independence for patients; respect for individual choice; and understanding of the diversity of individual needs (p. 34). These concepts appear in much contemporary nursing literature, such as the publications emanating from the Oxford and Burford Nursing Development Units. Enjoying a national reputation as centres of excellence, these units have claimed that their practice is 'the contemporary ideology of nursing in action' (Pearson 1988: 131). They are not typical of nursing today, but are often quoted as an example for others.

The philosophy of the ONDU (see note p. 23) was made visible by a large, colourful banner in the dayroom declaiming the words 'Growing in Partnership'. Quotations on the walls described 'partnership in practice': 'We listen to what the patient has to say and through . . . communication . . . we help him to become clear on his concerns around (his) particular treatment plan . . . he will clarify his own motivations' 'the nurses will aim to work in such a way that the patient becomes a partner who is actively encouraged to become an equal voice in decision making about his nursing and other therapies'. Some quotations were culled from America and British nurse theorists and ideas developed in publications, including a collection of essays by ward staff (Pearson 1988) and a research study (Pearson *et al.* 1988). Muetzel's definition of the nurse–patient relationship is typical of the general flavour: 'The power of nursing to promote healing lies . . . in this therapeutic relationship . . . a purposeful, supportive and healing association between two persons that is interactive and holistic' (in Pearson 1988: 89–90).

The essays take as their unifying theme primary nursing, a method of care delivery practised in the Oxford and Burford units and in other 'progressive' settings in the UK (Pearson 1988). According to Pearson, primary nursing is ideally suited to developing a close therapeutic relationship: 'Together a partnership can be created so that individual needs can really be identified and an individual plan of action constructed by both nurse and patient'. The nurse's accountability to the patient, and the authority she needs to 'begin to work in a professional way', lead to calls for greater autonomy for both; individually planned care and shared decision-making can only empower the patient if the carer has the power to allow the patient to enact those decisions – 'autonomy for the nurse means autonomy for the patient' (Pearson 1988).

Primary nursing is, however, seen as more than an efficient and effective mode of organizing and delivering care. Other contributors to the book argue that the close nurse–patient relationship which it promotes 'not only provides the milieu for expressing therapeutic methods, but has itself the potential to serve therapeutic effect' (p. 75). Nursing helps people to feel better as well as to get better, an outcome enhanced by the nurse's 'therapeutic use of self'. Intimate physical care, frequently delegated to junior or unqualified staff in the traditional division of labour, should be given by the primary nurse herself – because she can thereby offer physical comfort, but can also simultaneously give psychological and emotional support.

The belief that nursing is a therapy in its own right is explicated in a study of the effects of admitting patients to an experimental unit (ONDU) based on 'therapeutic nursing' (Pearson *et al.* 1988). The authors acknowledge that 'therapeutic nursing' is rarely practised in general hospitals, where nurses focus mainly on physical needs. Yet they find a growing belief that patients' needs can be met through 'meaningful interaction' within a holistic framework which helps them set realistic targets for change and supports them in reaching those targets. The nurse's role is seen partly as that of teacher or facilitator, enabling patients to marshal their own healing resources; involving patients as partners in care increases their knowledge and control of their health.

ONDU was explicitly established to enable a 'nursing ideology' to prevail, in the sense suggested by Williams (1974) of 'a pattern of ideas which provide overarching conceptions of social experience'. The nurses' ideas represent far more than a description of a method of care, or even a set of principles based on scientific knowledge, research findings or some other attempt to establish objective criteria. They also represent a value system, although those values are not made explicit beyond a vague sense of altruism. Moreover, the claim to be serving patients' interests masks many other considerations, which is no news to the sociologist but needs emphasizing because the interests of nurses and patients tend to be regarded – by nurses! – as identical. Although New Nurses claim to be acting in patients' interests, they are also challenging medical domination and seeking higher status for themselves.

Where does this idea of partnership originate? First, an attempt is made to locate it in a centuries-old tradition of women healers which predates nursing's domination by medicine and is now re-emerging from the shadows (e.g. Ersser in Pearson 1988). A second strand that also owes something to tradition is the advocacy of an individualistic one-to-one relationship, following the established model of a professional contract between expert and client. Yet the ideology also draws heavily on humanistic psychology, with its emphasis on openness, trust and honesty in the discovery of self through relationships with others. These traditions – medicine and psychotherapy – contain conflicting assumptions about power relations. To compound the complexity, the ideology has been influenced by consumer demands for changes in professional–client relationships.

The contradictions and confusions in the New Nursing's ideology do not, of course, discredit it. Like any set of beliefs it is a jumble of old and new, of ideas that are being assembled and may in future be discarded, of concepts from a number of disciplines. Even if it does not hang together well, it is distinguished from most nursing literature by its attempt to understand and justify as well as prescribe what nursing practice should be. It is also notable for some of its advocates' efforts to practise what they preach.

Partnership in practice

ONDU, which functioned between 1985 and 1989, was unique in the NHS. It contained 16 'nursing' beds for patients who were deemed to need intensive nursing but, having passed through acute biological crisis, no longer needed frequent attention from doctors. In any other hospital they would be found in acute wards. The admission of patients was ultimately determined by the senior nurse, who visited referred patients in the acute wards to assess their nursing needs.

Partnership was developed in practice at ONDU through measures that aimed to enhance the patient's autonomy, and recognize the individuality of patients and nurses. Interpersonal contact between nurses and patients was encouraged and seen as integral to the work. Staff attempted to offer patients genuine informed choice in their care, and to respect the choices made. One example among many was keeping patients' notes at the bedside: such measures seem modest but their implications are little short of revolutionary in challenging prevailing assumptions about the roles of patient and nurse.

The unit's staffing structure and work organization was shaped according to its nursing ideology, which regarded the traditional hierarchy and division of labour as obstacles to personal accountability to the patient (Pearson 1988). This lack of accountability was held not only to harm the quality of care, but to reduce the autonomy needed for the nurse to develop partnership with the patient and therefore, indirectly, to diminish the patient's power. Primary nursing was chosen as the method and philosophy for organizing nursing work as it appeared best suited to facilitating closer partnership with patients and greater autonomy for clinical nurses; the unit's primary nurses were called 'nurse practitioners'. Selected 'basic nursing' tasks often seen elsewhere as work for unqualified staff, such as bathing patients or helping them with eating, were being rehabilitated as professional work. The practitioner–patient partnership was also being staked out as professional nursing territory.

Each primary nurse had a small team of associate nurses also assigned to care for specific patients. This associate role, which had less autonomy than that of the primary nurse, was thought to be a 'learning post' suitable for newly qualified staff (including enrolled nurses) or part-timers. The logic of the ideology suggests that they will not develop such close relationships with patients, although they give a great deal of the care: does this mean the healing power of nursing still depends on hierarchical position?

Giving the primary nurse autonomy in the planning and delivery of care also meant a reformulation of the ward sister role. The unit had a senior nurse practitioner, formerly a primary nurse, whose role was to advise on clinical nursing, develop and support the staff, and manage the unit. She also co-ordinated its education and research programmes, and sometimes acted as an associate nurse.

The customary organization of nursing labour, whereby the bulk of direct care is given by junior and unqualified staff, had therefore been abandoned. The primary and associate nurses gave much direct patient care and it was seen as inappropriate for others to do so. The nursing auxiliary was replaced by a 'care assistant' whose role combined aspects of domestic and nursing work, including bedmaking, lifting patients, helping the nurse with procedures and clearing up, and testing urine – tasks said not to require the skills of a trained nurse. Their relationships with patients were not described as therapeutic partnerships; indeed the issue seemed not to be discussed, although they had their own subculture in which they made alliances with other ancillary staff and patients rather than with qualified nurses.

The relationship between nurses and care assistants mirrored the traditional doctor–nurse relationship, in which the nurse performs the (apparently) less skilled, routine, lower status work and the prime therapeutic relationship is that between doctor and patient. Care assistants on ONDU were allocated the most physically demanding, repetitive and mechanical work and were the lowest paid. The flattening of the nursing hierarchy was therefore only partial, and despite its unorthodoxy it preserved much of the traditional professional model.

One of the fascinations of ONDU was seeing these key debates in contemporary nursing playing out on its small stage. Another interesting factor was the research it had stimulated, since it is unusual if not unique for nursing in one setting to receive sustained attention. The most extensive study compared groups of elderly people for fifteen months in a randomized controlled trial; one group was nursed in the unit and the other in the district general hospital (Pearson *et al.* 1988).

The results supported the hypotheses that patients transferred to the unit for therapeutic nursing received better and more consistent care than their district general hospital counterparts; became more independent; were more satisfied with their nursing; were generally as satisfied with life; had a shorter average stay in acute care; and incurred lower average costs. A surprise finding was the statistically significant reduction in the death rate of ONDU patients while in hospital, compared with the control group. 'Nursing-led care has a positive effect on recovery, quality, satisfaction and mortality, which supports the study assumption that nursing in itself is a therapeutic force', the authors conclude.

The range of the study (and its political purposes) were such that it says little about nurse–patient relationships beyond a general conclusion that patients preferred the care they received at ONDU. Nevertheless the authors, who included the unit's previous and current senior nurses, felt able to argue that 'the new norms advocated by nursing leaders enhance therapeutic effectiveness' (p. 2).

Another smaller study looked at the relationships between nurses on four wards, including ONDU, which have different types of management structure (McMahon 1987). Arguing that the desire for autonomy for nursing ('which is being achieved by nursing allying with patients') leads to lateral or collegiate structures, McMahon sought to establish empirically whether they increase respect and trust or competition and conflict among nurses. He concluded that the choice of management structure made an appreciable difference to the 'power structures' of hospital wards. Staff interactions on ONDU exhibited fewer overt manifestations of power and were more likely to be social rather than functional. 'Primary nursing . . . resulted in the adoption of authority of knowledge rather than of position', he says. Positive results also emerged from a study comparing team nursing in a district general hospital medical ward and primary nursing on ONDU (Reed 1988). This found that primary nursing 'affords increased quality of care, a more coherent philosophy of nursing and increased job satisfaction for nurses' (p. 383).

These studies supported my own observations that ONDU provided good quality care using nursing initiatives which merit further scrutiny. Less cautious claims are fraught with danger, however, for reasons that the researchers themselves acknowledge. The studies face familiar methodological difficulties: finding reliable and valid measuring instruments; adequate sample size; dealing with observer/interviewer bias; and demonstrating external validity. Above all there is the problem of defining and controlling for extraneous variables. As Pearson *et al.* admit, their research was based on the assumption that the experience of being nursed in the unit was the independent variable: 'this could not, of course, be proved'.

ONDU's nurses achieved measurable success in putting into practice their ideal of partnership with patients, using a combination of practical procedures, changes in the division of labour, and the creation of a milieu in which patients felt physically and mentally comfortable and able to assert themselves. Given the difficulties of introducing major change in health care, this was an impressive achievement. Change on this scale is slow, however, and many issues remained unresolved. Most striking to me were those of persuading nurses to work in a way for which they had not been trained, and which challenged current practice among nurses and other professionals; the role of care assistants, including the unexplored dimensions of their relations with patients; and the nurses' relationships with doctors (by controlling admissions and relegating doctors to a consultancy role, these nurses largely sidestepped the power struggle that such changes would provoke within a more conventional setting). By no means least problematic was the patient's role and expectations.

The attempted transformation of the nurse–patient relationship is not a simple matter of one-to-one communication, but has implications for these and other issues; like a house of cards, it is impossible to shift one element without disrupting the entire structure. Equally it is impossible to understand the dynamics of the nurse–patient relationship, and the issues involved in changing it, without looking at the many factors that help to shape it within and beyond the walls of the ward.

Constraints on nurse–patient partnership

ONDU inevitably had its share of problems, and the hostility of some doctors eventually led to its closure (see note, p. 23). Most if not all its difficulties are experienced by other nurses attempting similar reforms, and some are intensified in settings where the therapy is not nurse led. ONDU's experience therefore merits attention for its broader relevance as well as its intrinsic interest.

The New Nursing says the one-to-one relationship between practitioner and patient is the foundation of good nursing. Developing such relationships in the current climate faces many material and structural barriers, not least the difficulty of recruiting and the cost of employing sufficient numbers of trained staff. Even supposing such barriers could be surmounted, the question remains whether most nurses and patients wish to develop relationships of this type. Furthermore, can the New Nursing work in settings where nurses are not highly motivated like those at ONDU – do most nurses want to be New Nurses? Sociological studies can shed some light on both questions.

Patients and professionals

Sociologists have highlighted the misapprehension that professionals and users of health services share the same world-view, goals, and concepts of health and illness (e.g. Freidson 1970). As an organized division of labour nursing has goals that cannot be assumed to be identical with those of patients. Illness behaviour and an understanding of illness as social conduct have been probed in many studies; as a recent review concludes, lay people have a complex body of health knowledge and beliefs which is rooted in the social context of their daily lives (Calnan 1987). This almost inevitably leads to Freidson's 'clash of perspectives' between professional and patient.

Finding out what lay people want from nurses could help to determine how far the New Nursing is profession – rather than patient – led. For example, patients in one study judged the quality of nursing by its 'emotional style' (Smith and Redfern 1989). The focus of the nurse–patient relationship does address an area of great importance to patients – but a desire to be treated with warmth, kindness and sensitivity does not necessarily mean all patients want close relationships of a quasi-psychotherapeutic kind. Although the New Nursing ideology draws on humanistic psychology, it does not address the major assumptions underlying formal psychotherapeutic practice, such as the agreement between professional and client on the goals and parameters of the relationship. The immediate concern of patients is likely to be relief from pain and discomfort, rather than a meaningful relationship in which they can discuss their personal problems. Their physical needs bring them into intimate bodily contact with nurses, sanctioning actions normally permitted only to parents or lovers, if at all. This relationship has different boundaries, suggesting that subsuming it in a psychotherapeutic one may be problematic.

The New Nursing's use of this model also neglects consideration of how the part played by faith or belief might make an hierarchical relationship beneficial for patients (Parsons 1951). Anthropological evidence shows that the special powers attributed to healers in many cultures assists cure; Western medicine is likewise a symbolic belief system in which 'effectiveness' depends partly on people's expectations (Young 1976). This suggests that demystifying the relationship might actually reduce its therapeutic potential.

Ungerson's analysis of relationships between carers and cared-for raises further relevant but underexplored questions (1983). She argues that the 'dirty work' of physical caring is seen as women's work in society's sex-role stereotyped division of domestic labour. Professional women carers are likely to bring the motherhood model to their relationships with physically dependent patients, which suggests further barriers to partnership in the way both nurses and patients conduct the relationship. The power relations work at another level: most nurses are women, so will male patients accept them as equal partners in care?

As Ungerson concludes, 'The sexual division of labour and its relationship to tending tasks has a central place in any analysis of the caring relationship'. This key point has tended to be underplayed, however, by the supporters of the New Nursing. Pearson, for example, notes the gender issue (Pearson 1988), but explicitly distances his concept of good nursing from the 'unskilled intuitive feminine acts of a mother' while deploring the 'follies and prejudices' of a society which 'decries nursing as simple "women's work"'. This might be expected of a group seeking higher status; the strategy is sometimes all too traditional in its attempts to escape the shaming association of nursing with female domestic labour.

The evidence that patients want partnership with nurses of the type being advocated is, therefore, rather mixed and needs more consideration. But what of nurses themselves – do they want to work in this way? Recent studies illustrate the gap between professional rhetoric and nurses' own priorities and preferences.

Nurses' views of nursing

Buckenham and McGrath (1983) investigated everyday, routine social inter-actions in hospital wards and interpreted that world through the eyes of the nurse. Although their study was conducted in Australia, the similarities of the nursing culture suggest its findings are relevant to the UK. Focused, semi-structured interviews elicited attitudes to four 'critical incidents' which obliged nurses to choose between two sets of behaviours, exemplifying the roles of handmaiden or patient advocate. Although the nurses supported the professional rhetoric of putting the patient's needs first, all except one failed to do so in 'reality' even when it exposed the patient to serious risk: 'You know what should be done, but it's a bit different when you're actually there', said one (p. 64). Their primary allegiance was to the professional health team, and they would only act as an advocate if this did not jeopardize team membership.

The study concluded that the qualified nurse saw her main function as assisting and supporting the doctor, a deep loyalty that was related to her desire to stay in the team. The price paid for membership was subordination. Despite what they were taught in the classroom student nurses arriving in the wards were immediately presented with an image of themselves as subordinate members of a subordinate division of the health team. Internalization of this image could then create a downward spiral of reduced self-esteem and acceptance of the handmaiden role. 'The consistency of the derogatory responses that the nurses perceive the doctors to be directing to them serves to influence both their self-concept and their behaviour' (p. 59).

Melia's study of the occupational socialization of nurses in Scotland in the late 1970s reveals a similar landscape (Melia 1987). From informal interviews with student nurses, five analytic categories emerged to describe how they 'fitted in' to ward life:

1 focusing on how they learned the rules to pass as workers;
2 how the work was organized and performed;
3 their dual learning/working role;
4 the implications of their transient position;
5 their communication with patients.

Many interesting points emerge from Melia's fruitful accounts; of special interest here is the organization of the work. The ward's main business was seen to be 'getting the work done', with work presented to the students as sets of routines. The ideal of patient-centred care was eroded by many factors including staff shortages, lack of time, and the bureaucratic management system employed by most ward sisters; a mixture of organizational constraints and the emotional safety of routine work led to task-orientated nursing. According to the unwritten rules, talking to patients was not 'real work'; even when time was available, students should not talk to them but should 'look busy' performing some mechanical task. After three years doing the work, being a staff nurse conferred the sought-after power to supervise it instead.

All this suggests that students would have to rebel against the system in order to build partnerships with patients. They accepted 'a subordinate position for nursing in relation to medicine in the area of communication' (Melia 1987: 88), an acceptance demonstrated in many other areas including the way they talked about nursing. 'Real nursing' described the technical/medical aspects of the work, while 'basic nursing care' was low status, uninteresting, and could be (and was) done by anyone. The students took their lead from the medical profession in determining which areas of care they were most prepared to value; these became 'real nursing' (p. 136).

A similar pattern emerges in Smith's study, in which the students preferred 'technical nursing' and valued it as learning material: 'meeting patients' emotional needs was recognised as neither work nor learning material (unless legitimised by a medical speciality). Although they associated high quality with wards where nursing's affective components were both visible and valued by qualified nurses, they did not think they needed to be taught how to do 'emotional labour', but could meet patients' affective needs through the interest in people which had brought them into nursing (Smith 1988).

Smith argues that unlike technical nursing, affective and physical aspects are taken for granted as women's natural work. Keyzer (1988) also discusses New Nursing theory in relation to gender issues. He argues that frameworks such as

Henderson's, which claim to be patient-centred and to challenge the traditional power of nurse and doctor, can in reality be used to reinforce existing power structures. A truly patient-centred model would challenge the boundaries between the roles of the doctor, the nurse, and the informal female carer: 'it is unlikely that such a model . . . would be welcomed by those whose power it seeks to remove', he says.

The implications for nursing

Consideration of the professional–client relationship suggests that partnership is by no means straightforward. There is also a lack of clear evidence that patients want the kind of relationship advocated in 'therapeutic nursing'. Furthermore, the accounts of nurses' views indicate that major changes are needed in their occupational socialization and in the organization of hospital work if they are to practise in this way.

All these studies are reminders of the world beyond the ward, and imply a host of other factors that will influence the spread of this ideology. The division of health care labour, from doctors to care assistants, still rests on traditional inequalities in gender, race, and education, so tinkering with its internal boundaries will make little difference without broader social change (though it can be argued, of course, that the New Nursing is itself a symptom of changes in the social composition of nursing, and nurses' expectations and aspirations). The current state of the NHS, with budget cuts and problems in nurse recruitment and retention, suggests that new models of care may only take root if they are cheaper, or employ unqualified staff. Moreover, the evolution of the NHS into a managerial culture is antipathetic to the professional model of practice being proposed.

These and other factors prompt the question 'why now?', because this does not seem a promising time to propose such changes. Over a decade ago Carpenter predicted that managerialism in the NHS would lead to a revival of the professional model and a search for clinical solution to nursing's status problem (Carpenter 1977). His predictions were accurate, but it is not yet clear whether the New Nursing is simply another manifestation of old-style professionalism, or whether it contains the seeds of a more radical reorientation of nursing towards true partnership with patients. Looked at another way, the reform proposals could even be interpreted as primarily a struggle for occupational survival (Salvage 1988).

More challenges are posed for the analyst by attempts to categorize the leaders of the New Nursing, usually on the unspoken assumption that the categorization is an aid to understanding motivation. Carpenter described three main groups in nursing: rank and file, new managers and new professionals (clinical specialists outside the hierarchy who undertake delegated medical work). Melia adds 'academic professionalizers', found mainly in academic circles and somewhat distant from patients (Melia 1987). 'They seek to achieve autonomy for nursing by elevating the status of "basic" or "primary" care . . . to promote a style of nursing founded on "nursing theory" . . . rather than . . . tradition and medical dominance', she says.

Even this classification is too simple. Today's clinical leaders are neither ivory tower academics nor privileged specialists, although some have created positions with considerable autonomy. Two characteristics are probably significant: some have studied in higher education after a period in clinical practice, and a disproportionate number are men. Their understanding of health care is increasingly sophisticated; to accuse them of pure élitism seems too crude. Melia asks whether the theorists' intellectual activity is undertaken for altruistic reasons concerning patient welfare, or whether it is a means of achieving academic and professional status – but she acknowledges that professional status brings the power needed to improve care.

Melia is surely right to imply that the New Nursing's agenda moves far beyond a concern to improve patient care. The New Nursing is not a parochial issue in clinical nursing, but it is (among other things) an occupational strategy seeking higher status, rewards and power for nurses (or some of them). My own study focused on how it lays claim to authority by articulating and developing the interpersonal, affective aspects of nursing which are said to have therapeutic power. The movement also makes other claims in other ways. It claims authority from the undervalued skills and expertise of nurses (which supports its demands for better and continuing education); through its use of scientific research; and through its responsiveness to society's health care needs. These are large claims and they require careful scrutiny.

The leaders of the New Nursing need to guard against the seductive assumption that empowering nurses is the route to empowering patients. It is inevitable that they should wish to raise the status of clinical nursing, but they should be wary of assuming that this in itself will benefit patients. Exploration of other key issues, such as the impact of gender on nursing and the division of nursing labour, also needs to be encouraged. Otherwise there is a danger that the reform movement will either fall into the traps of traditional professional élitism, or fail because it reproduces current power relations in health care.

The avoidance of these uncomfortable issues is marked, however, in the New Nursing literature and discussions – and this could be counterproductive. Unless they are willing to scrutinize these issues, and their own beliefs and practices, the New Nurses will miss an important (and perhaps unique) opportunity to develop ways of nursing which will significantly improve patient care. A lack of critical thinking will also diminish their ability to achieve their goals. Their vision can never be realized unless they have a strategy for reaching it, and they cannot plan such a strategy without a clear assessment of all the forces which are likely to help or hinder them.

Policy analysts and researchers have a major role in ensuring that the awkward questions continue to be asked. In particular, the studies cited here demonstrate the value of the sociological perspective in generating critiques. Yet, despite the fertile ground that nursing offers to sociologists, 'medical' sociology and feminist sociology have largely passed nursing by, even though the issues are germane not only to health care but to society in general. The nature of modern professionalism, occupational socialization, the organization of work and the role of women – are all key societal issues for the 1990s and beyond.

To end on a positive note, the achievements of one setting where the ideology of the New Nursing underpinned practice suggest that positive change can occur. Although the ONDU's successes cannot be ascribed to any one cause, they are none the less important for that. If this new style of nursing does lead to better care and more satisfied staff, it deserves close attention from health care managers and policy-makers. It is their responsibility to remove the constraints on working in this way which lie within their power, just as it is the responsibility of nurses to tackle those factors that fall within their remit and sphere of influence. The implications of the issues which the New Nursing raises are central to the future of nursing, and therefore to the future of health care.

Note

1 The ONDU (Beeson Ward, Radcliffe Infirmary) was closed by Oxfordshire Health Authority in March 1989, after this study was completed – despite its high quality, innovative work and excellent standards of care, reflected both in research and in patients' comments. Following intensive lobbying by nurses throughout the UK, who were angered at this attack on an acknowledged centre of nursing excellence, the health authority agreed in principle to establish nursing beds elsewhere in the district, though at the time of writing no location had been identified. The reasons for the closure merit a study in their own right and, in the context of this chapter, demonstrate the immense obstacles nurses face when they attempt to work as autonomous practitioners. (For brief accounts see Salvage 1989; Pembrey and Punton 1990.)

2

The nursing workforce: Aspects of inequality

Kate Robinson

Kate Robinson's chapter is a further forceful critique of new professional reforms in nursing. Looking specifically at primary nursing, Kate Robinson speculates on the course that primary nursing may take in the context of a workforce separated into core and peripheral sectors. She begins by taking a critical look at the composition of the nursing workforce, drawing attention to its highly stratified nature. Sexual and racial divisions within the NHS, she suggests, mirror divisions within the wider society. She then assesses the impact that primary nursing is likely to have on the composition of the nursing workforce and the distribution of opportunities within it. Kate Robinson's conclusions on this subject merit serious attention. She suggests that the implementation of primary nursing may result in the creation of an élite 'core' workforce of primary nurses who are dependent on a larger 'peripheral' workforce of associate nurses and support workers. Not only, argues Kate Robinson, will career opportunities for those seeking to move from the peripheral to the core workforce be severely circumscribed; but those primary nurses with domestic commitments may find themselves on a downward career progression from positions within the core to those within the peripheral workforce. The division of nursing

into two increasingly separate workforces, Kate Robinson concludes, will exacerbate existing inequalities
between men and women, married and single women,
black and white, thereby reinforcing sexist and racist attitudes in society as a whole.

Introduction

The nursing workforce is clearly an important element in UK society because
it fulfils a number of caring functions which are currently dealt with in the
public domain. However, the size of the workforce also makes it an important
component of the social order. The composition and structure of the nursing
workforce reflects the apparent 'natural' order in society, but it also reinforces
it. Changes in that composition and structure may in time be reflected in the
way things are ordered in society as a whole.

The importance of accurately predicting changes in the nursing workforce
in relation to particular strategies of change were highlighted in the Project
2000 exercise, a large part of which was concerned to predict the shortfall of
labour if nurses in training became supernumerary. However, in this chapter I
want to explore the relationship between another recent nursing innovation –
primary nursing – and the nursing workforce, and to propose that evaluation
of such innovations should include a consideration of the predicted impact on
the workforce as a whole.

The anatomy of the nursing workforce

The days of chief nurses having to lay the lists of nursing personnel on their
office floor and count them (Robinson and Strong 1987) are over. Computeriz-
ation of payrolls has meant that the total numbers of the nursing workforce
employed in the National Health Service (NHS) are much more readily available. Figures are held centrally as well as within the employing authorities. The
clear message of these figures is that the nursing workforce is a major
component in the employed population in the UK, and a particularly significant
part of the female workforce.

The nursing and midwifery staff (NHS) total in England in 1987 was
410 633, in Scotland in 1989 it was 74 829, and in Wales in 1988 it was 27 918
whole time equivalent (wte)[1]. In other words, if you said 'roughly half a million'
you would not be far wrong. This compares with a total workforce in 1986 of
just over 21 million. That is to say, about 1 in 40 of all employed workers in
this country is working as a nurse. The distribution of this workforce does not
correspond, however, to the distribution of the total population (National Audit

Office 1985; Gray 1986). The health service in Scotland, for example, employs more nurses than would be expected on the basis of population (Gray 1986). Nurses work in a number of different settings. In England, for example, 77 per cent of nurses worked in hospital settings in 1987. Of course, there are also many nurses employed in the independent sector but as yet the NHS remains the largest employer.

The workforce is highly stratified. Apart from the obvious categories such as qualified and unqualified staff, there are a range of distinctions within these categories. For example, a group of qualified clinical nurses on one ward can be in posts graded from C to I; movement between the grades depending on movement from one post to another. About 1 in 3 nurses works part-time, and the proportion of part-time workers increases in the lower reaches of the grade hierarchy (Gray 1986).

Nearly half – 45 per cent – of the total UK workforce is female, but within the nursing workforce the figure rises to approximately 90 per cent. However, although the majority of the nursing workforce is female they are not evenly distributed throughout it. In England, for example, 1 in 6 full-time staff is male; the proportion for part-time staff is 1 in 72. The findings that large numbers of women, but not men, in nursing are working part-time reflects the importance of part-time female labour in the workforce as a whole; 43 per cent of the female workforce works part-time. Studies have also found that, even in comparison with their full-time female colleagues, the number of men in the higher positions in nursing is disproportionately high (Carpenter 1977; Davies and Rosser 1986). In Davies and Rosser's study, fieldwork in two districts, one rural and one urban, demonstrated that:

> In both settings, however, and despite the small number of men, men were found disproportionately represented in the higher grades. They comprised fully 37 per cent of those in posts of nursing officer and above in the rural district, and some 13 per cent of those in comparable positions in the city district. Patterns by speciality, service/education differences, and low proportions of men in Enrolled Nurse (EN) grades and as auxiliaries, and their virtual absence from part-time work at any grade, are further features.
>
> (Davies and Rosser 1986)

What of the ethnic mix within nursing? Nursing certainly recruits from ethnic minority groups and the Department of Health collects information on the birthplace of NHS staff but does not publish it; neither is data published on the ethnic groups within the health service (Gordon 1988). However, ethnic monitoring does seem to be increasingly carried out at district level.

A number of studies offer some data on the jobs held by black nurses (Torkington 1987; Baxter 1987). They indicate that black nurses are over-represented in lower grades such as EN grades. They are also clustered in the less popular specialities such as mental health and mental handicap nursing, and under-represented in work in the community such as health visiting, and popular specialities such as paediatrics.

The physiology of the nursing workforce

What are the processes that produce this nursing workforce? The responsibility for constructing the nursing workforce rests with the local employers rather than with the NHS. This is succinctly stated in the Report of the Comptroller and Auditor-General (NAO 1985):

> Department of Health and Social Security (DHSS) delegate to health authorities responsibility for detailed planning and control of nursing manpower subject to the constraints of available finance and manpower targets . . . DHSS accept responsibility for ensuring that nurse manpower planning is properly carried out by health authorities as part of their overall planning, and for scrutinising and where necessary challenging authorities' plans, but consider it neither practicable nor appropriate for the department to plan the demand for, and supply of, nursing manpower nationally.
>
> (NAO 1985: 2)

It must be said, however, that the government controls a number of factors such as pay and conditions which will crucially influence the availability of recruits to nursing. It also has ultimate control over the entry gate to the profession through control of the system of registration.

Within district and area health authorities, responsibility for human resource organization may be delegated to a number of different levels – units, sub-units and, increasingly, wards. Within a structure that delegates budgets, including the human resource budget, to ward level, decisions about the composition of the workforce and the recruitment of staff will be dealt with at that level. Local nurse managers will therefore make decisions on skill mix according to their perceptions of nursing need.

Such recruitment will, of course, be bound by local policies on the recruitment of staff, which will in turn be constructed according to legal and traditional definitions of 'good practice'. However, there is still ample evidence of discriminatory processes at work in recruitment within the health service; it is these processes, combined with the racism and sexism within society as a whole, that produce the skewed picture of human resource distribution presented in the previous section.

Racial discrimination

Evidence of racism has been provided by a number of research studies (Hicks 1982; Baxter 1987; Torkington 1987). Baxter concludes, from her study in Manchester:

> Black nurses experience special difficulties at every stage of their entire career. Their problems are concentrated mainly in the areas of recruitment, deployment and promotion.
>
> (Baxter 1987: 25)

Black nurses reported being channelled into enrolled nurse training and discouraged from attempting conversion to first level, and channelled towards mental health and mental handicap nursing, regardless of their preferences. They reported being denied access to conversion courses. In work they were channelled towards the night shift; Baxter quoted a nursing officer: 'They love the night shift. It must fit in with their way of life' (Baxter 1987: 36).

Pearson (1987) quotes figures from a review of the ethnic composition of staff in South Derbyshire which showed that black nurses are over-represented in low-grade positions. They made up a disproportionately large number of enrolled nurses and auxiliary nurses. Pearson writes:

> In summary, 97 (49 per cent) of 198 Afro-Caribbean nurses were employed as auxiliaries, but only one was a clinical nurse manager. This pattern of racial inequality of access to senior positions is consistent with that reported in other studies of London and Liverpool.
>
> (Pearson 1987: 26)

Sexual discrimination

The different paths taken by men and women in nursing has been a source of debate and division as well as the subject of a series of research studies. The first study to come out of the Edinburgh University Nursing Research Unit – the first nursing research unit in the UK – was Hockey's *Women in Nursing* (1976) which explored the experiences and career paths (or career dead-ends) of female nurses. At about the same time Brown's DHSS sponsored study of male nurses' careers was reporting '. . . male recruitment is a valuable source of nurses capable of taking positions of responsibility' (Brown 1975: 99).

During the 1970s the possibility of male domination within the nursing profession was being pointed out by a number of commentators; see, for example, Dingwall 1972 and 1979; Nelson 1976; Carpenter 1977. Dingwall (1979), for example, argues that nursing may gradually be developing into a male-dominated occupation, just as primary teaching and social work have. This is not merely a sociological concern. Nelson (1976) writing in the *Nursing*

Mirror 'Personal Viewpoint' page under the heading 'Male domination ahead?' commented: 'In the past we relied entirely on single women, and when their numbers were reduced we looked to men to provide the kind of hours worked by single women'. Dingwall, building on Carpenter's analysis, argues that the advantageous position of men can be linked to the domination of scientific expertise within the health service. Men rather than women, it is believed, are able to think and act in the kind of rational scientific ways necessary for functioning in the new management structures in the health service. The Salmon Report emphasized the importance of these attributes within nursing – the report has therefore been seen as a 'male nurses' charter' (Austin 1977). The consequences of the introduction of management thinking and structures include the splitting of the workforce into three groups – a skilled or semi-skilled group of workers and two élite groups, the nurse clinicians and the nurse managers.

The first group – the 'proletarian' nurses – includes the large number of nurses who are working part-time. They do not in general include large numbers of men. Davies and Rosser (1986) have described the processes of sexual discrimination working within the health service. They concluded that there was no active consideration of the working patterns of women. Specifically, women with domestic commitments were seen as potential problems, and job criteria worked against those who took career breaks or could not be mobile:

> Again and again those we interviewed would set men and women in different camps. Women, either all women or some women, they would say, really did have other goals and commitments. Some people went so far as to say it was morally wrong for women with small children, for example, to try to hold down a demanding job. Others just saw women with children or who might have children as a 'hassle' in management terms, as potential absentees. It would not be too strong to say that they subscribed to doubt about the viability of women as workers.
>
> (Davies and Rosser 1986)

The evidence from Davies and Rosser's study was that there was 'no support at all for the notion that men were career minded and women were not'. In fact neither men nor women reported wanting to move away from contact with the patient.

A more recent study (Mackay 1989) focusing on nurses' accounts of their own experience supports the proposition that married nurses and nurses with domestic responsibilities who work part-time find working life difficult:

> Part-time nurses are considered as very much second-class members of the team, given no opportunity or encouragement to embark on further studies or courses. This appears to be management policy. (Staff Nurse)
>
> (Mackay 1989: 79)

The picture painted above is of a profession in which racial and sexual discrimination is commonplace. An additional dimension needs to be considered in relation to gender, which is marital status; single women may be able to maintain a status in advance of their married sisters who are seen as having the threat of pregnancy and child care hanging over them.

A reformist strategy

However, it is important to say that there have been attempts at reform. Interest has focused rather more on the sexual question than the racial one, which has been the subject of more localized concern. The concern about the position of women has been particularly strong because of recent concern over the lack of recruits to the nursing workforce. In 1986, Trevor Clay, then General Secretary of the RCN voiced his, and by implication the organization's, concern in a speech at the Royal Institute of Public Administration:

> The largest waste of resources in the NHS is the loss of qualified nursing staff. Three years of training and several years' experience are lost because management have passively accepted existing attitudes to women and their pattern of work.
>
> (Clay 1986: 20)

His proposals included additional workplace facilities for small children, additional opportunities for part-time working and enhanced return to practice programmes. However, he was concerned that opportunities for part-time work must be supported by a commitment to career progression for part-time workers:

> But with it must go clear commitment for regarding these individuals, and encouraging them to regard themselves, as still having potential for promotion. In nursing this is not the case, and women who return part-time quickly lose their place on the ladder, being overtaken by other, usually single or male, nurses.
>
> (Clay 1986: 22)

The issue of Return to Practice has been taken up by the government which has funded an open learning course presented by the Open College. The problems of creating opportunities for part-time workers to make a contribution relevant to their skills have been explored on a smaller scale, through job share or flexitime schemes. Standard shift patterns can be modified at ward level (Fitzgerald 1990) and doubtless such changes are taking place in many parts of the country. Job share schemes, however, seem to be relatively rare. The nursing press has described a number of such schemes (Buchan 1987; Shuttleworth 1988) and it is clear that their advantage for the job holders is that they can retain the advantages and security of a full-time post at a higher grade while working part-time. Many of the nurses currently working part-time on low grades are undoubtedly capable of working at higher grades – as anyone who has been in contact with bank nurses is aware. Lathlean, who evaluated a job share scheme in London (1987) recommended that more job share schemes should be established by health authorities. However, there seems to be little interest in such a general movement, which would have to be quite substantial if it was to redraw the picture of discrimination towards married women.

The reformist effort related to racism in nursing has tended to focus on areas with a high black population. For example, West Lambeth Health Authority embarked in 1985 on an extensive strategy of positive action designed to increase the numbers of black nurses in the health district which has a large black population. An Equal Opportunities Working Party, which included representatives from local government and equal opportunities organizations as well as the health authority, established an access course linked to the School of Nursing for the local population. It also aimed to encourage black nurses into the acute unit. Such efforts do not commonly, however, link action against racism with action against sexism. Black women recruited into nursing in West Lambeth Health Authority will face the same sexual discrimination as white women; the policy may operate largely in favour of black men in preference to black women.

Professional reformism: Primary nursing

I want now to look at a particular innovation in the organization of nursing care – primary nursing – and to consider what changes, if any, the introduction of primary nursing is making to the composition of the workforce.

Primary nursing is considered to be both a system of organizing nursing care and a philosophy of nursing. Philosophically, it is based, like so much of contemporary nursing rhetoric, on the ideals of individuality and personal development fostered in America in the 1960s. The organization allied to this is the allocation of one primary nurse to each patient for the purposes of assessing their needs, prescribing care and evaluating care. This nurse will normally also be expected to deliver much of the care herself. However, in order to supply the 24-hour care conventionally offered to people in hospitals, the primary nurse heads a team of other nurses – known as associate nurses – who deliver care when the primary nurse cannot. They are expected, however, to administer the prescribed care rather than take diagnostic or prescriptive decisions on their own behalf.

The ideas of primary nursing seem to have been promoted in the UK from about the late 1970s (see, for example, Lee 1979) and were associated with the development of nursing practice units, particularly Burford (Pearson 1988). Primary nursing is now being promoted by many of the influential bodies within nursing. For example, it has been endorsed by the Chief Nursing Officer for

England and the Minister of State for Health (Department of Health 1989a). The Director of Nursing at the King's Fund has made the promotion of primary nursing a major focus of development work (see Chapter 1).

Since Manthey (1980) first described primary nursing, there has been a wealth of research attempting to demonstrate its effectiveness. Here I will rely mainly on reviews of that literature (Giovanetti 1986; MacGuire 1989; Bond *et al.* 1990). Despite the plethora of studies, we do not know whether the innovation of primary nursing generally improves outcomes according to a number of measures. This is for two reasons; the first, that much of the research is poorly designed and executed: 'While there is a voluminous literature about primary nursing, much of it is anecdotal and descriptive' (Bond *et al.* 1990); second, because those studies that are methodologically satisfactory have not produced sufficient or sustained evidence of change in outcome. This is hardly surprising given the complexity of distinguishing the effects of nursing inputs from those of other inputs. The outcome measure most commonly found in the literature is patient satisfaction, but staff satisfaction has also been used as an important indicator of value – perhaps because the introduction of primary nursing is a response to staff rather than patient dissatisfaction. An outcome measure that has not received significant attention is the consequences for the composition of the nursing workforce. With a major innovation in the way any job is organized – the introduction of an assembly line, for example – one would expect a major focus of concern to be the consequences for the size, distribution and opportunities of the entire workforce. This aspect has been largely ignored, including, as far as one can see, by the major nursing unions.

What are those consequences likely to be? The following discussion must proceed largely by speculation, partly because the research data is not available and partly because primary nursing is as yet only a small part of the organization of the workforce and may take some years to work through – assuming of course it is not superseded, as is indicated by some anecdotal data from the USA, by case management systems before it achieves full supremacy.

In order to contrast the role of primary nurse with that of associate nurse I have taken the following description from Tutton's (1986) account of primary nursing in the ONDU at the Radcliffe Infirmary. While this unit was by no means typical, being a 'nursing beds' unit, the development of primary nursing in Oxford had been a model for its development in many other parts of the country:

> *Primary nurse* – Primary nurses take a case load of eight patients each, carrying full responsibility and accountability for their care. They assess, plan, implement and evaluate this care, leaving a written care plan for associate nurses to implement in their absence. If a change in this plan of care is needed, the nurse practitioner is contacted and will either give a verbal instruction or visit the unit.

Associate nurse – These are trained nurses, often part-time, who carry out the care planned by the primary nurse, under whom they are divided into teams. They have a case load of eight patients.

(Tutton 1986: 39)

We can supplement Tutton's description of primary nursing in a ward with a study of primary nursing in a community hospital (Bond *et al.* 1990). In this situation, 'Birchover' ward had three primary nurses – all full-time staff. Each was assisted by two associate nurses either full-time or part-time and two or three part-time nursing auxiliaries. The primary nurse role, as portrayed by Bond *et al.* (1990), is one in which there is every encouragement and opportunity for the primary nurses to improve their skills. They participated in the multidisciplinary team meeting and it is clear that they expected to be accorded status and respect by the doctors and other colleagues.

Bond *et al.* report that the organization of primary nursing was difficult to achieve, requiring some reorganization:

. . . by reducing the number of organisational units to three, varying shift patterns and staff grades, and *bringing in casual labour on a regular basis* the staff creatively achieved primary nursing in organisational terms.

(Bond *et al.* 1990: 22, emphasis added)

The normal work pattern for a primary nurse is full-time day shiftwork. For example, Sear and Williams (forthcoming) specify a minimum of 34 hours, although MacGuire (1989) considered that a minimum of 20 hours per week is acceptable. (Of all part-time workers just over half work under 21 hours per week (Department of Employment 1989).) However, it is clear from Tutton's account that primary nurses may have to work unpredictable hours in excess of their arranged shift; in the event of a nursing emergency: '. . . the nurse practitioner is contacted and will either give a verbal instruction or visit the unit'. MacGuire's specification is similar: 'In exceptional circumstances she may be called in to see a patient when she is not on duty'. This requirement is currently being reviewed in at least one district with a view to offering open ended contracts of the 'to work all hours necessary to fulfil the duties' type.

There is evidence that this places an unacceptable burden on some nurses. Another study of primary nursing in a community hospital (Johns 1989), using a qualitative methodology to explore the impact of the introduction of primary nursing on the hospital culture, found that invasion of personal time was a practical issue for some nurses, as can be seen in the following data extract:

The primary nurses were equivocal about being contacted at home. The two single primary nurses felt they should be (contacted at home):
'I've said I want to be rung at home . . . a lot of people here don't agree with that, they feel you should be totally separate at home and that you are too involved in your work if you want to be called up at home, so they haven't.'

... The other two primary nurses supported the prevailing culture. One remarked:
'When I'm at home I like to think I've got a private life as well. ... I don't think it would be fair on my husband if I can't go out in case somebody rings up from the hospital. I think there has to be a limit as to how much you can deal with ... and just to switch off when you get home.'
... Both these primary nurses had considerable family commitments and felt that family life was their primary role outside work life.

(Johns 1989: 88–9)

Core and periphery

The work of Carpenter (1977) and Dingwall (1979) reported earlier provides the basis for the view that the nursing workforce consists of three segments – the proletarianized workforce, the élite clinical nurses and the managers. The introduction of primary nursing can be seen as a victory for the élite clinicians who have defeated the nursing managers at the cost of admitting a large number of primary nurses to their ranks. Within primary nursing the management of nursing is relegated to a subsidiary supportive position. Decision-making – of standards, skill mix, and nursing goals – and not just of individual patient care issues is seen as the prerogative of the team of primary nurses, albeit with the support of the ward sister/charge nurse.

However, what of the majority of the workforce, that is, those who will act as associate nurses and support workers? Clearly the primary nurses will be the élite core of nurses; trained to a high level both academically and in terms of key skills such as assertiveness, they will expect to be participating as equals in innovative schemes, research work, and further development work. The district that cannot offer them these rewards for the commitment they are offering will find itself without a core of able nurses to run the service. But such work rewards are, of course, scarce resources. If they are offered to the élite group there will be little left over for full-time associate nurses and even less for part-time and bank staff – those groups that have already experienced massive discrimination. The gap between the two groups will widen and consequently will become harder to bridge for those part-time workers or full-time associate workers who might want to move to primary nursing positions.

What sort of workforce will have been promoted by the introduction of primary nursing? Looking at the UK workforce as a whole, Walby (1987) explores a model of a flexible workforce developed by Atkinson (1986). The model proposes that the workforce is increasingly divided into a 'core' work-force and a 'peripheral' workforce. The core consists of skilled workers, employed for long periods on secure contracts with good promotion prospects.

The periphery consists of semi-skilled or unskilled staff on insecure contracts and frequently employed part-time with few career prospects. Atkinson argues that the distinction between the two types of labour is increasing the segmentation in the labour market. The employers favour increasing the peripheral labour forces as a response to employment protection legislation, because part-time labour is cheaper per hour than full-time labour, and because peripheral labour may be numerically flexible, that is, employers can vary the amount of labour they employ at short notice.

Walby tests the general model of the core/peripheral distinction against the gender structure of the workforce and suggests that the use of an extensive peripheral workforce to enhance the flexibility of labour use may be segregating the workforce along gender lines. However, the length of the working week is used as the mechanism to justify it – and thus to avoid the penalties of anti-discriminatory legislation. But how closely does the model of a flexible gendered workforce correspond to the post-primary nursing scene? It is clear from the discussion of primary nursing above that the introduction of primary nursing may depend on the existence of a peripheral workforce. Furthermore, some workers who are currently full-time primary nurses may be forced out of that role by the necessity of a commitment beyond the working shift. Unable to foresee a return to primary nursing status, they would soon join the ranks of the peripheral workforce – a career break might see them within the peripheral workforce as part-time workers.

Is the distinction between core and periphery gendered? The discussion above would indicate that, *at present*, it is not consistently segregated on gender lines. For one thing, there are not currently enough men to constitute an adequate core within a primary nursing system; only one full-time worker in six is currently male. The data – which is as yet inadequate – would seem rather to support a distinction between, on the one hand, men and single women, and on the other hand, married women and women with children. While married women without children may be able logistically to sustain a position in the core workforce, there is little confidence among their managers in their ability to do so, at least until their prime child-bearing years have passed. What of black nurses; what is their place in the flexible workforce? We know that they are over-represented within night duty and in the lower grades – elements of the peripheral workforce. And the processes of discrimination described above would clearly operate to keep black nurses, and particularly black female nurses, out of the core workforce.

An unholy alliance?

The NHS had long been a battleground between the interests of the professionalizing tendency within nursing and the interests of the employers. Within nursing the most recent debates have been about occupational closure;

the professionalizers arguing for a high-status single portal, while the management have been concerned to open the entry gate to sustain the levels of nurses necessary to staff the service. However, on the organization of the nursing workforce it would appear that the interests of the professionalizers and those of the employers may coincide. While the employers are concerned with the potential costs of a high-status élite profession, their worries are ameliorated by the creation of a flexible cheap peripheral workforce. This workforce consists currently of nurses qualified to both registered and enrolled nurse status and support workers. As the support workers' training acquires academic status and the worth of the qualified nurses' qualifications becomes eroded by time and comparison with Project 2000 Diplomates and degree nurses, it is difficult to see the distinction between the types of peripheral workers being sustained. This could force the cost of such workers downwards unless powerful union pressures oppose such a downward drift, and it is hard to see where such union pressure might come from.

It is important, in such situations, to avoid overuse of conspiracy theories and I would not like to suggest that the senior clinical staff who are experimenting with primary nursing are involved in a plot with management to create a peripheral flexible workforce. But it seems to be clear from evidence supplied by some of the few studies of primary nursing that offer qualitative data (Johns 1989; Bond *et al.* 1990) that the creation of the highly skilled nursing élite necessary to primary nursing is being achieved at the expense of the majority of the workforce. Or, to put it another way, is primary nursing the vehicle through which the clinical nursing élite are consolidating a position as a profession based on just a part of the nursing workforce?

MacGuire (1980) proposed a possible future in which 'male managers face female workers'. Ten years later, do we see control being wrested from the nurse managers, partly through the clinician's control of the new nursing curricula where scientific rationality is being replaced by phenomenological approaches to caring? The clinical élite is not wholly male, but it consists largely of those unencumbered with competing demands on their time. The innovators might think it worth considering, however, why the introduction of primary nursing is being supported by a government that is not committed to professionalization within the health service – it is always worth looking closely at the motives of one's bedfellows.

Moreover, the female segment of the professionalizers might be wise to cast a glance at their male colleagues who are disproportionately represented within the core workforce. If the core was ever required to retract, as it might if financial pressures force a move to a case management approach where the primary nurse deals with assessment and the management of the 'case' and leaves most of the nursing to less expensive nurses, then, given the processes of discrimination that have remained essentially untouched, the female component of the core would undoubtedly be most at risk.

However, that is not my main concern. Nor is the position of many of the workers in the peripheral workforce, although I am dismayed that the optimism of the equal opportunities legislation cannot be translated into any real gains. My real concern is with the image that a workforce divided, at least to some extent, on racial and gender lines offers to the country as a whole. It is an image that reinforces rather than challenges beliefs about the position of women and black people in our society and which therefore damages everybody's health.

Note

1 Unless otherwise stated the statistics are taken from: *Health and Personal Social Services for England 1989*, DoH 1990a; *Scottish Abstract of Statistics 1989*, Scottish Office 1990; *Health and Personal Social Services for Wales No 16 1989*, Welsh Office 1990.

3

Nurse manpower planning: Role, rationale and relevance

Jim Buchan

Jim Buchan's chapter describes nurse manpower planning as pragmatic, management-led attempts to identify and address the actual and potential problems of mismatch between the supply of and demand for appropriately-qualified nursing labour. Jim Buchan argues that nurse manpower-planning is a function rather than a discipline and that it will always be dependent on inexact methods. The demand side of the equation is always subject to numerous variable factors, manipulation of the supply side lies much more in managers' hands, but balancing the two requires policies for which there is little evidence on costs or benefits. It appears therefore that the key issue is not identifying potential solutions to supply–demand imbalances, but rather establishing which policies are likely to be effective and efficient.

Introduction

'Manpower Planning' is a term which, for many readers, will sit uneasily in the context of determining staffing requirements in nursing. 'Manpower' is a singularly inappropriate label for an occupation that is predominantly female – in the NHS 93 per cent of nursing staff are female (DoH 1990b).

Whilst the phrase 'manpower planning' can be regarded as a misnomer for a female-dominated occupation, the substitution of other titles such as 'human resource planning', 'workforce planning' or 'personnel planning' can have drawbacks, because such phrases can suggest a less quantitative and broader perspective within the personnel function than that concerned directly with matching supply and demand. This chapter therefore uses the phrase 'manpower planning' because it has a common currency in describing a discipline or sub-discipline, and generally summarizes the issues and methods to be discussed, but the chapter is written in the full acknowledgement that the phrase is inappropriate for a female occupation. The extent to which the inappropriateness of terminology revealed by the use of the phrase 'manpower' may be linked to inappropriate manpower planning techniques being adopted for nursing staff will also be examined in the chapter.

The role of manpower planning

The role of manpower planning is to effect the balance of demand for staff with its supply – to ensure that sufficient (but not over-sufficient) numbers of appropriately qualified personnel are available, in the right place and at the right time to match the demand for their services.

Nursing manpower planning, as a function in the NHS, links service planning and personnel management and is closely linked with planning for other staff groups, such as doctors and the professions allied to medicine.

On the demand side, the function of manpower planners is to assist in determining the appropriate number and mix of nursing staff and other employees, for a given catchment population, number of hospital beds or planned number of cases.

On the supply side, the function of manpower planning is to assist in determining future requirements in the supply of nursing staff, assessing the comparative magnitude of various 'flows' of staff into and out of the service (*from* training, *to* career breaks etc.) and working with personnel specialists in developing appropriate personnel policies to keep these flows in the required balance, therefore best meeting the demand side requirements for staff.

The manpower planning function can therefore be summarized as having three main elements:

1 Assessing how many, and what type, of staff are required (demand side).
2 Identifying how these staff will be supplied (supply side).
3 Determining how a balance between demand and supply can be achieved.

Each of the three elements makes use of specific methods and techniques, which are best examined by considering in detail each element. It is important, however, to appreciate from the outset that the role of manpower planning can only be properly realized if its three elements are integrated and if, in turn, the manpower planning function itself is assimilated within the broader objectives of the organization, in terms of its planning and personnel strategies. Manpower planning cannot be properly conducted in isolation from service planning and personnel management, and as such it cannot be readily identified as a discrete discipline. (Indeed if it is, it is likely to be isolated rather than integrated.) It is, or should be, an identifiable and adequately resourced function within the overall strategic and planning arm of the organization.

The phrase 'organization', within the healthcare sector, may reflect a single employing unit such as a hospital, or can be used to describe other operational levels – within the NHS these are at unit, district, regional and national level. Manpower planning takes place at each of these levels; its role and priorities varying in each. At the local level, the priorities will relate primarily to day-to-day planning and allocating staff to workload. At the strategic level, the priorities will be linked to longer term issues of supply and demand, such as ensuring sufficient recruits are entering nurse education, to meet expectations of future demand.

The next three sections will consider in detail each of the three elements of manpower planning outlined earlier (demand side, supply side, and matching demand and supply), drawing on relevant examples from nursing in the NHS, and elsewhere.

Demand side

The assessment of need – answering the question 'how many nursing staff do we need' is fundamental to nurse manpower planning. It is a question to which there is no single 'right' answer – the answer will vary, depending on the methodology or methodologies adopted to determine demand. This lack of specificity can lead to criticisms that manpower planning is not worth the effort – that it is an inexact science producing inexact results. The counter-argument is that manpower planning is not intended to produce precise results. Its function is to assist in the planning of resources by enabling management to develop systems and controls which enable the organization to make better use of its internal labour market and to identify the position of the organization in the wider labour market context and react flexibly to changes in the external labour market.

As Branham noted 'criticisms of forecasting and planning often imply that there is a choice between undertaking manpower planning and not doing so. In practice the real choice is whether to be systematic in planning or to be swept along by events. Decisions are made whether or not they are planned, but even rudimentary planning will improve the quality of decisions made' (Branham 1982).

More than 300 000 nursing staff are employed in the NHS. The size of the nursing workforce, the recurring paybill costs and initial training costs mean that nursing accounts for a significant element of expenditure, in a highly labour-intensive organization. As such, planning to ensure effective use and deployment of nursing staff has a financial, as well as operational, imperative. The tension between two measures of demand – 'how many nursing staff do we need?' and 'how many nursing staff can we afford?' is ever present, and it is one role of manpower planning to assist in determining the second measure and so (in theory at least), influence the level of funding available, and decisions on affordability.

The demand side element in manpower planning can encompass a whole range of issues. Assessing the demand for nursing staff can include the following:

1 assessment of 'need';
2 measuring workload;
3 setting establishment levels;
4 managing deployment to cover 'peaks and troughs';
5 job analysis and competency mapping;
6 skill mix, grade mix and role overlap;
7 absence control;
8 use of 'bank' nurses, temporary and short-term contract staff;
9 use of computerized establishment control systems, rota planners, etc;
10 clinical audit, quality audit and quality assurance (i.e. measuring input *and* outcome).

At the simplest level, the 'need' for healthcare provision can be based on an assessment of the catchment population to be served by the organization (be it a single hospital or a national health service).

This need may be linked to targets for future improvements in the provision of healthcare, which will have direct implications for the assessment of demand for staff. Such targets may be related to, for example, the World Health Organization (WHO) 'Health for All by the Year 2000' criteria (Shipp 1989 – review of demand estimation in a number of WHO affiliated countries), or may be linked to other desired improvements in the provision of healthcare services, such as the reduction in waiting lists. Whilst such target setting can serve a useful purpose in providing clear objectives and in concentrating the organizational mind, there is a danger that, if the targets are regarded as unattainable 'ideals' they will not be accommodated within the strategic planning function, and therefore the implications for staffing levels will not be considered. The implementation of the White Paper (DoH *et al.* 1989b), with subsequent delineation of 'purchasers' and 'providers' within the NHS, will lead to a greater emphasis on realistic and measurable targets, which will be contractually set.

Estimating the demand for nursing staff can be approached on one of three levels:

1 Using staff/population ratios, as measured by the judgement of likely need for healthcare.

2 Using staff/population ratios, according to *actual* historical met demand for healthcare (there may also be unmet demand, e.g. waiting lists).
3 Using staff/workload ratios, as measured by the workload generated, in terms of hospital beds, or bed occupancy rates, or caseload size, etc.

Whilst the use of population profiles (i.e. 1 and 2 above) can act as a preliminary indicator of demand for healthcare, there are a number of limiting factors which must be considered (Waite forthcoming). These include:

1 The impact of 'cross boundary' flows of patients/clients between population catchment areas. For example, central London hospitals provide a service to many patients/clients who do not reside within the catchment population area; these hospitals also attract patients from elsewhere, because of their teaching hospital expertise.
2 The impact of differing population profiles, e.g. an 'old' profile population will have a markedly greater demand for healthcare than will a 'young' population.
3 The role of other governmental (e.g. local government), independent (e.g. nursing homes) and voluntary bodies (e.g. hospices) in providing healthcare has to be accounted for if the demand for the services of nursing staff in the NHS is to be accurately assessed.
4 Variations in the extent of horizontal and vertical overlap between the work of nursing staff and the work of other groups of healthcare workers (e.g. professions allied to medicine, junior doctors, and support workers) has to be considered in assessing the demand for nursing staff.
5 Variations in work organization, such as shift patterns, shift overlap and whether patients/clients are visited individually, or seen at health centres will impact on the actual demand for services, and therefore on the demand for certain types of nursing staff.
6 Differences in the budgetary priorities ascribed by different organizations to different care groups and staff groups will lead to different levels and 'mixes' of nursing staff and other groups of health workers being employed.

It is evident that there are a number of limitations in using such ratios, which should be made explicit to avoid misunderstanding or misinterpretation. The use of population/staff ratios can, however, provide some indicator of likely demand for services, and can allow some comparison of variations in the level of demand between different units, regions or countries. For example, geographical variations in the population/nursing staff ratios were revealed in the report of the National Audit Office (NAO 1985, see also 1990) which demonstrated that the number of nursing staff per 100 000 population varied between 75 (Oxford Region) and 173 (Mersey Region) in the NHS.

The use of formulae that link the demand for staff with financial and demographic projections is often characterized as the 'top down' approach to manpower planning. The top down approach, if it does not take account of local circumstances, including the factors outlined above, has limited relevance. In reality, in most situations some elements of the 'top down' approach are combined with local factors and local judgements – and in some situations, computerized establishment setting and workload allocation systems – (the 'bottom up' approach) in determining future nurse staffing requirements.

Many of the shortcomings of nursing population ratios can be overcome by utilizing this 'bottom up' approach to estimating demand which was outlined above – that of determining the staff required per unit of workload, in terms of number of beds, bed occupancy levels, caseloads, or other measures of need.

There are four main types of approach to the measurement of workload experienced by nursing staff:

1 Outcome can be measured, and related to the 'input' of staff.
2 A detailed work study approach can be used, to assess timings of activities.
3 The current range of staff/workload ratios can be measured. 'Norms' can be determined, and 'high' and 'low' outliners identified.
4 The professional judgement of practitioners can be utilized to assist in establishing the appropriate staffing levels required to meet measured workload.

There are benefits and drawbacks to each of the four options. Measurement of outcome (option 1) represents the 'ideal' approach, but at the time of writing there is no general consensus on the appropriate methodologies and criteria for assessing outcome and quality of care provided. Utilizing the work study approach (option 2) is comparatively time consuming and expensive, and inflexible – changes in staffing levels or workload would require the study to be replicated. Assessing current 'real' staff/workload ratios and setting 'norms' (option 3, e.g. the 'Aberdeen' formula) allows for variations in the ratio to be identified, but does not indicate what is the ideal ratio. The professional judgement approach (option 4, e.g. the 'Telford' approach) provides a simple 'user friendly' tool for local managers and professionals, but provides less detailed information on the activities of staff (Bright 1985; Malin 1986).

Assessing future demand for nursing staff will always be an inexact science, because it is not possible to identify or measure accurately the impact of the variable factors which will impinge on future staffing requirements (not least the future availability of funding). The longer the timescale of assessment, the greater will be the margin of error, but the lesser will be the requirement for detail in projections.

Supply side

The supply side of the equation, assessing the future supply of nursing staff, is both more readily assessable over a longer period of time, and more open to control, because of the key role the NHS plays in training nurses.

The near monopsony[1] position of the NHS, as a purchaser of the services of nurses, is reinforced by its monopoly role as the only provider of basic level training of nursing staff and the major provider of post basic training. It therefore acts both as the arbiter of the magnitude of the 'flow' of new nurses, by determining the number of training places provided, and as the market leader in terms of determining how many nurses will be employed, and at what level of pay it will employ these staff (see Yett 1975 for a discussion of the monopsony effect in USA healthcare labour markets).

The future supply of newly trained nurses can be measured with some degree of accuracy, because the time lag between entering nurse education and qualification enables a three year forward projection to be made. The current magnitude of other inflows, due to nurses returning from career breaks, or from other forms of employment, and outflows due to retirement, career breaks and 'wastage' to other forms of employment can also be quantified, using available data, trends in that data and an assessment of the impact of external labour market factors.

Ensuring the supply of sufficient nursing staff to meet demand is a subject of considerable concern, because of the much publicized demographic decline in the source of 'traditional' recruits to nursing (female school leavers) and widening employment opportunities for these potential recruits (National Economic Development Office 1988). However, regional variations in the extent of demographic change and varying levels of unemployment at a local level mean that the impact of school leaver decline will vary between different localities – therefore management led solutions to demographic decline will also have to vary in different localities (Waite and Pike 1989).

The trend in the number of entrants to nurse training has been one of reduction in recent years (although figures for 1989 suggest a modest increase), but much of the fall in numbers can be accounted for by the phasing out of training for the second level of the register (i.e. enrolled nurses) which is one result of the implementation of Project 2000.

Project 2000 – the move of nurse education into the higher education sector, with supernumerary status for nursing students – will in itself have major implications for the future supply of nursing staff, both in terms of their quality and quantity. One of the arguments utilized in achieving governmental support for the funding of Project 2000 was that the current 'traditional' form of training had high levels of wastage, and that supernumerary status and a broader, college based education would lead to improved retention of students.

Modelling current and future supply of nurses from training was one of the manpower planning techniques utilized in assessing the likely impact of Project 2000 (Hutt *et al.* 1985; Price Waterhouse 1987). These models had to rely on assumptions on future wastage rates. Modelling assumptions that wastage from training will reduce as Project 2000 is implemented may prove to be optimistic if student nurses avail themselves of the easier opportunities to transfer to other courses within the higher education system, or if 'reality shock' occurs (if the nature and reality of nursing in the work environment is perceived to be different from that which has been instilled during the three year training period).

Assessing the supply of 'new' nurses (i.e. those who have entered the professional register for the first time, having completed basic training) represents only part of the exercise. Other sources of inflow available to the employer have to be evaluated. These sources are nurse returners, re-entering the labour market after a period of economic inactivity, individuals returning to nursing from non-nursing employment, and nurses entering or re-entering the UK labour market from abroad (Welsh Office 1987).

The requirement for any nurse who wishes to practise to register their professional qualifications with the UKCC enables an overall picture at national level of the UK 'pool' of nurses to be assessed, and also allows an assessment of the magnitude of some of these flows into and out of that pool.

'New' entrants to the register (i.e. those coming from schools of nursing and entering the register for the first time) represents the inflow which can be measured with the greatest degree of accuracy and can also, at least in theory, be most readily influenced by policy (i.e. by increasing or reducing the number of training places). In recent years there has been a declining trend in the number of new entrants entering the register year on year. This is partly due to the phasing out of enrolled nurse training but also reflects a reduction in the number of student nurses qualifying for the first level of the register. The underlying reason or reasons for the decline in the numbers entering training for first level registration is not known, but widening career opportunities, a continuing reliance on female school leavers at a time of demographic decline, and the poor 'image' of nursing as a career have all been cited as likely factors.

Detailed information on the number of re-entrants – nurse 'returners' – is not available (in teaching women returners are a more important source, numerically, than are new recruits) but policy attention is turning to this source of supply as the number of 'new' recruits has declined. Increasing female participation rates and shortening career breaks have been characteristics of women's employment in the UK over the last three decades, but this has been mainly due to individual choice rather than to supportive policy. However, in the NHS nursing context there is now the beginnings of a supportive policy framework, with the establishment of the RCN/Open College 'Return to Nursing' learning package to update skills and restore confidence, and the Whitley Council agreement for a five year 'managed' career break for NHS staff.

Greater manpower planning emphasis on the female 'returner' as a source of recruits is not limited to nursing or the NHS. Many other sectors, particularly service industries, have identified the expanding pool of 'mature' women as a replacement source for the dwindling number of school leavers. The identification and implementation of personnel policies to best tap this 'pool' has received considerable attention in recent years (e.g. Metcalf and Leighton 1989). Some commentators have expressed a desire that the establishment of greater equality of opportunity in employment, which is the end result of many of these policies, should not be merely a temporary phenomenon linked to current labour market pressures but should mark a permanent shift to more equitable employment practices.

The most detailed manpower planning research on nurse returners and potential returners was conducted in Scotland (Waite *et al.* 1990) and revealed that considerable numbers of nurses currently on career break were considering returning to NHS employment at some point in the future. The research also underlined that a lack of flexibility in working hours, absence of childcare, and downgrading of those who had occupied promoted posts, were regarded by many individual ex-nurses as major obstacles to return. Less detailed, but similar research has been conducted in Northern Ireland (Centre for Health and Social Research 1990); there are no comparable data at a national level in England (but see Nessling and Boyle 1990, for a replication of the Scottish study in an English NHS region).

Another source of supply of, and destination for, NHS nurses is the non-NHS healthcare sector. Until recently the role of the independent sector was often not considered explicitly at national or regional level when NHS manpower planners were assessing nurse supply, but there have been moves to build in the effect of the independent sector when modelling future nurse demand and supply. Research indicates that the independent sector is a destination for more nurses leaving the NHS than a source of nurses joining the NHS (Waite *et al.* 1989) and there has been considerable growth in the numbers of nurses employed in the independent sector in recent years (Buchan 1990b). The growing influence of the independent sector as an employer of nurses has led to recommendations that the NHS and non-NHS employers be more closely involved in planning and funding the supply of nursing staff (NAO 1990).

It should be evident that any attempt to assess or plan the supply side has to be underpinned by the knowledge that the vast majority of nursing staff are female, and that the characteristics of the nursing workforce as a predominantly female workforce will have an impact on the supply side behaviour. One important factor is that much of the 'wastage' from nursing employment is not permanent, but is linked to career breaks for family reasons; many female nurses who leave nursing will wish to return at a future date, and many of these returners will be looking for part-time and flexible working hours employment, so that they can sustain domestic commitments. The oft-heard statistic that 30 000 nurses are 'leaving the profession' every year is misleading, suggesting as it does the end of a career, rather than a break in career.

It is necessary to take due account of different lifecycle stages in assessing the career and domestic commitments of all employees, particularly in a culture that continues to place particular responsibilities on females during the child-rearing years. If an employer is to make the most cost effective use of comparatively 'expensive' employees (i.e. those that it has invested time and money in training), particularly at a time of tightening labour markets, it will have to accommodate the demand for career breaks and the changing priorities of employees at different stages of their lifecycle (Bevan *et al.* 1990; Davies 1990).

The full implications of the nursing workforce being a female workforce, in terms of provision to meet demand for career breaks, part-time employment and flexible hours, have not always been properly appreciated by those responsible for nurse manpower planning. Whilst the implications of these issues have been recognized by some for decades and some planners have attempted to accommodate them, it is only recently that a more systematic approach to managing career breaks, improving career opportunities for part-time nurses, and establishing greater flexibility in hours of employment has been generally promoted.

Cynics will point to managerial self-interest at a time of tightening labour markets as the major factor in the promotion of a more systematic approach. Realists will welcome these moves as a positive step forward, recognizing that they are partially the result of broader societal and cultural changes. Those responsible for planning current and future supply of nurses will be primarily concerned with ensuring that the broad issues identified above are transferred into practical personnel policies.

Matching demand and supply

The previous two sectors have considered separately the role of manpower planning in evaluating demand, and in assessing supply of nurses. In reality, neither exercise can be conducted in isolation from the other, or from the effects of other factors relating to wider policy considerations and funding availability. It was noted in the introduction that manpower planning is at best an inexact science, and the match of supply and demand will never be exact, because the context in which the planning process is conducted is ever changing, with some changes being more predictable than others.

What the planning process does achieve is to highlight areas of specific concern in the short term (which will require immediate remedial action) and areas of potential concern in the longer term (which may be avoided, accommodated or addressed by adopting new personnel policies or altering current policies). The former can be characterized by 'reactive' action, the latter by 'proactive' action.

The available indicators on the demand side of the equation suggest that the demand for healthcare in the UK over the next decade is likely to grow. The underlying reasons for the projected increase in demand are well documented and relate to demographics (a growing population, with more elderly people), advances in medical practice and technology, the impact of 'new' diseases and infections (e.g. HIV/AIDS) and changes in public expectations of the healthcare system.

As noted previously, such projected increases in demand (which in the case of some factors such as population growth can be measured with some accuracy) will not necessarily be met in totality; it is likely that in the future, as now, some demand for healthcare will be unmet, some postponed.

Supply side indicators, as outlined previously, point to increasing difficulty in maintaining the supply of 'new' nurses from traditional sources. Coupled with the projected increase in demand for healthcare, this has led to much concern about 'nursing shortages' (i.e. a shortfall in supply, in relation to demand). The extent to which the shortfall can, or should be met by increasing the supply of nurses represents a core area of current debate between govern-ment, the DoH, the professional bodies and organizations, and trade unions.

The debate is about identifying how best to meet the increased demand for healthcare (the fact that there is increasing demand is not disputed), and centres on the determination of the appropriate level, mix and allocation of resources (financial and staffing).

In this context, the role of the support worker is regarded by some as the 'solution' to the nursing shortage. The support worker will be recruited from a wider pool, will require less time and finance to train, and will be less expensive to employ. The end result would be a shift in the balance of skill mix, with a lower proportion of registered nurses, and a higher proportion of support workers and nursing auxiliaries. (The working relationship, short term and long term, between support workers and auxiliaries remains unclear at the time of writing, Buchan 1990c.)

There are other potential solutions to the 'nursing shortage'. Four broad areas where manpower planning research indicates that there is scope for management action are as follows.

Maintain/improve school leaver intake

To maintain or improve its 'market share' of school leavers, the NHS would have to adopt strategies that may be costly, and will have no guarantee of success, given that other employers will also be gearing up to recruit from a finite and declining resource.

Improving the 'image' of the service amongst potential recruits (e.g. who are at school, as is happening with the current NHS advertising campaign) is one means of addressing the issue, but the cost can be high and the benefits difficult to assess.

The most direct approach to improving the recruitment of new school leaver recruits is to enhance relative initial pay rates significantly. The NHS is likely to be at a disadvantage in competing in labour markets on pay terms with private sector health organizations and service industries who have greater flexibility and financial resources, and can more readily bear or pass on the costs of an increased paybill. However, any marked decline in the relative position of initial and potential NHS pay rates could also undermine the positive benefits of any campaign to promote the image of NHS employment. The recent implementation of a clinical grading structure for NHS nurses and the implementation of Project 2000 may, once firmly established, provide a more attractive employment package for potential recruits than the hierarchical structure they replaced.

One further possibility is to 'widen the entry gate' to basic training for nursing. The main source of school leaver recruits are those with five or more O levels, and one or two A levels. If entry requirements were 'loosened', this would provide a greater potential pool of recruits. It would also, of course, have possible implications for the quality of new staff being trained and entering the service.

Improve recruitment from alternative sources

From a nursing perspective, any source other than young white female school leavers can be regarded as 'alternatives'. Men, ethnic minorities and mature entrants, are all underrepresented in nursing.

As previously noted, attracting a greater number of 'mature' entrants to training provides one possible source of recruits. For such a policy initiative to be effective, it will have to be recognized that the requirements and objectives of mature entrants may differ markedly from those of an 18-year-old recruit – for example, the provision of part-time training and/or childcare facilities may act as incentives for some mature entrants. It will also have to be borne in mind that these 'mature' entrants will also be targeted by other employers – in particular the projected growth in the service sector suggests that the NHS will face strong competition when attempting to recruit in 'older' labour markets. The comparative attractiveness of NHS nursing pay rates, post basic training availability and career opportunities will have to be subject to constant review.

However, research conducted by the Institute of Manpower Studies (IMS) on the Scottish nursing labour market (Waite *et al.* 1990) suggests that recruiting and training mature entrants can be cost effective – in terms of the number of years' employment which mature entrants 'give back' to the NHS, they do not compare unfavourably with younger entrants.

Improving the rate of re-entry of nursing staff who have left NHS employment is another policy option which requires careful consideration. The recent 'Return to Nursing' project launched under the aegis of the RCN is one example of an initiative designed to raise awareness of the potential for employing returners.

One other potential 'non-traditional' source which cannot readily be assessed in detail is the recruitment of trained staff from other countries – particularly in post 1992 Europe. The extent to which such freedom of movement will increase inflows *or* outflows of staff cannot be readily evaluated, and in the near future there will continue to be professional and language barriers which may militate against large-scale emigration. At present flows of nursing staff between the UK and continental European countries are at an insignificant level (Buchan 1990a).

Improving retention

Scope for improving retention exists both in improving the initial entry rate of those who have successfully completed training for the profession and in reducing wastage rates of qualified staff.

IMS research on NHS nurses suggests that increasing staffing levels, providing support and occupational health counselling, improving pay and conditions, and providing career opportunities for part-timers would assist in improving retention (Waite *et al.* 1989). The complex interaction of pay, job satisfaction, career prospects and non-work issues means that there is no 'quick fix' solution. Raising pay levels is certainly not the only answer, although the implementation of clinical grading may have had a net positive effect in encouraging retention in clinical areas (Buchan *et al.* 1989).

A number of non-pay initiatives relating to improving retention have been recommended for health authority action by the DoH. These include job-sharing, childcare facilities, and flexible hours provision. It is difficult, however, to establish a national overview of the extent to which these initiatives have been transferred into practice at local level, and even more difficult to evaluate their relevance or success, for little data are publicly available.

In particular, there is little hard evidence to facilitate an evaluation of the costs and benefits of using any one initiative, or 'package' of initiatives, and an associated danger that the absence of information may lead to policies inappropriate to local conditions being applied.

Improve staff utilization

The fourth area in which a number of policy options exist is improving staff utilization. Improving deployment of the staff is one means of coping with increased workload. As noted previously, current skill mix – within nursing and in relation to other NHS staff, qualified and unqualified – is also an area that requires detailed consideration. Issues relating to the quality of care provided have to be balanced against cost effective use of available staff, and one area requiring attention, both on cost and quality of care grounds, is the use of unqualified support workers.

The role of part-time staff is another area that provides potential for a more effective use of current resources. Many nursing staff work part-time because they have other, non-work related commitments. Part-time posts have, until recently, been generally regarded as 'pairs of hands' posts, in nursing and in other NHS professions. The attitude has been that only full-time staff can display the career commitment required to work in more senior and promoted posts. Whilst this attitude is beginning to change, partly as a result of the requirement to improve retention rates, it should be noted that relegating and marginalizing experienced staff to non-career posts because they wish to work or return to work on less than a full-time basis is also a less than effective use of available resources.

There are a whole range of possible policy options to consider when addressing the issues surrounding the matching of supply and demand. The appropriate mix of policy options for any one employer will depend on their staffing requirements, their available resources, and the conditions of the labour markets in which they are, or could operate. The real challenge to management and manpower planners is not identifying potential solutions to recruitment and retention difficulties (these are well documented), it is identifying *which* solutions are effective and appropriate to their circumstances and objectives.

Note

1 Monopsony – where there is only a single purchaser of goods or services.

4

A general manager's view of contemporary nursing issues

Chris West

Chris West's chapter looks at the main trends and events that have affected the organization and management of nursing from the mid 1950s until today. Placing his historical account within the context of wider social and economic change, Chris West identifies nursing's triumphs as well as its losses. The latter part of the chapter is devoted to a discussion of the way forward for nursing in the face of current political and managerial reforms. His message is clear. In the search for cost-effectiveness in health care the nursing labour force will change both structurally and quantitatively. The rewards for high performers will be off-set by the losses experienced by those who for whatever reason cannot compete.

In exploring the policy issues facing nursing from the perspective of a district general manager, it is important to look retrospectively at the main trends in the NHS and in society which have occurred over the past two to three decades.

The pattern of hospital management, through hospital management committees (HMCs) and boards of governors, was confirmed in 1954 by the Bradbeer Report which recommended that hospitals should be managed by a triumvirate of a hospital secretary, the chairman of the medical staff committee and a matron (CHSC, MoH 1954). However, hospitals were only components within the remit of HMCs which invariably covered more than one hospital and the group secretary of the HMC, or in the case of boards of governors, a clerk, house governor or secretary to the board of governors, had clear executive authority over the hospital secretary and frequently, by implication, over the matron.

The publication of the Salmon Report of the Committee on Senior Nursing Staff Structure in 1966 (MoH, SHHD 1966) sought to create a managerial structure for nursing that ensured the representation of the profession at employing authority level and thereby unquestionably enhanced the status of nursing throughout the service. Initially it was intended that there would be a phased implementation of 'Salmon' with a pilot scheme to test and evaluate the concepts and recommendations. However, in 1968 the DHSS took the decision to implement the Report's recommendations throughout the NHS.

Many administrators welcomed the Salmon Report. Some undoubtedly for the positive reason of strengthening the status of nursing, of giving due recognition to the importance of effectively managing nursing services, and (almost as a precursor of resource management) recognizing the value of involving staff with a clinical background in the process of managing resources. Other administrators, however, may have been slightly more cynical and simply saw the advantage of strengthening the clinical knowledge and power base in the administrator/medical divide so that the doctors could be taken on more effectively. I suspect, furthermore, that a number of key administrators resented the loss of their clear dominant position and did not welcome the introduction of the Salmon Report at all. Neither did most medical staff who found the new terminology difficult to understand and nurses' new managerial roles difficult to cope with. Also, since to many there was no apparent improvement in the quality of care or availability of resources at patient care level, many consultants were actively hostile to the Salmon Report and in 1990 continue to grumble about it!

The Briggs Report published in 1972 (Briggs 1972) sought to raise the importance of nurse education and the management of resources devoted to this function. In addition, the committee recognized the importance of changing the traditional ways in which student nurses were recruited and trained, and some of its recommendations were to be extremely appropriate in addressing the recruitment problems arising from demographic changes in the late 1980s and 1990s – for example, the establishment of mature entrants' training programmes. Furthermore, the action that was taken in 1989 in introducing the reforms of nurse education contained in Project 2000 (UKCC 1986a) can be traced back to the Briggs Report. It is regrettable that the timescale between proposal and delivery seems to be so long in the NHS.

The publication of the 'Grey Book' (Management Arrangements for the Reorganized National Health Service) in March 1972 (DHSS 1972) confirmed the already strengthened position of nurse management within the NHS. It consolidated the position established by the Salmon Report and also its equivalent in the community health services, the Mayston Report (DHSS *et al.* 1969).

The chief nursing officer at district, area and regional health authority level was given organizational equality with chief officers in the other NHS management functions, such as finance, administration, community medicine and, at district level, on district management teams, along with the representatives of general practitioners and consultant medical staff. Given that the chief nursing officer at district level was responsible for managing 50 per cent of the labour force in the district, and over a third of the budget, nursing had moved into a very powerful position.

The 1970s started with such promise. At the end of the 1960s the revenue growth rate to the NHS was increasing by up to 5 per cent per annum in real purchasing power; cash limits had not been heard of; the Resource Allocation Working Party (RAWP) (DHSS 1976), with its effect of redistributing resources away from hospital services in London had not yet been published; and the capital programme throughout the NHS had increased dramatically.

In 1973 the level of expenditure on the capital programme in the NHS reached a point that was not exceeded until the 1980s with the return of a Conservative government. All seemed to be set fair, particularly for nursing, with money flowing into the NHS in ever-increasing volumes, and a major reorganization taking place designed to bring together all aspects of the service within one organization. The allocation of even more resources to an integrated service promised to fulfil the aspirations of many people associated with or working in the NHS.

However, off stage events were occurring that would shatter such gentle aspirations. In October 1973 the Organization of Petroleum Exporting Countries (OPEC) in response to American policies in the Middle East following the then most recent Arab/Israeli war, decided to double, and subsequently treble the price of oil exported to the industrialized world. Furthermore, in response to rising inflation in the UK, the cabinet decided to remove £2 billion from public sector expenditure. Capital schemes were cut and, at the very time when the NHS needed the experience of its most senior staff, many took early retirement under the personnel policies published to facilitate the introduction of the changes set out in the Grey Book (DHSS 1972). In January 1974 the National Union of Mineworkers, having banned overtime working in the autumn of 1973 as a response to the Heath government's pay policy, decided to stage an all-out strike to break the prices and incomes policy of the government of the day. A general election was called. The Conservative party lost and in late February the Labour party was reinstalled as a government without an overall majority. Barbara Castle, as the newly appointed Secretary of State for Social Security, made it clear that whilst she did not support the changes that were taking place in the NHS, she nevertheless felt it impractical either to defer or to alter them.

The earlier application of a prices and incomes policy had had another effect on the NHS in October 1972. The traditional link between the pay awards for ancillary staff in local government and those in the NHS was broken and as a result, for the first time, staff working in the NHS took industrial action. This was a major change in culture in the service, and following the assumption of responsibility for the re-organized service by regional health authorities (RHAs), area health authorities (AHAs) and district health authorities (DHAs) on 1 April 1974, staff involved in the direct provision of clinical care to patients also took industrial action in pursuit of pay claims. Nursing staff, para-medical and scientific staff all took industrial action and in 1976 so did a number of medical staff. The reduction in expenditure on the capital programme, the very significant reduction in revenue growth, the introduction of cash limits, and in 1976, the publication of the RAWP Report (DHSS 1976) combined together with the complexity of the new management arrangements for which little training had been given, resulted in many parts of the service being left without effective leadership. A delegation from the RCN and the British Medical Association (BMA) went to Downing Street to press the Prime Minister for an additional £500 million to be given to the NHS. The government's response was to set up a Royal Commission.

The much greater restriction on funding and the reduction in growth for both capital and revenue (particularly when compared with the growth rates recently experienced in the late 1960s and very early 1970s), together with the increased power of trade unions, particularly those representing ancillary staff, such as National Union of Public Employees (NUPE) and Confederation of Health Service Employees (COHSE), caused the more articulate lobby groups within the NHS to press for the abolition of AHAs, the restoration of matrons and additional funding to be provided for the service. The low state of morale within the NHS and the loss of any sense of pride by some staff resulted in widespread industrial action in the winter of 1978/79. In May 1979 there was a general election and the Conservative government returned to power.

With the appointment of a clinician as Minister for Health the nursing profession and, to an even greater degree the medical profession, enjoyed a close rapport with and high esteem from the government. Further organiz- ational change occurred in 1982 with the implementation of the Conservative government's proposals in the consultative paper *Patients First* (DHSS and WO 1979); AHAs and sectors were abolished but the principle of consensus management at district and regional level was retained. One of the first acts of the Conservative administration in response to pressure from the nursing profession was to reduce the number of hours in the standard working week for nurses to thirty seven and a half hours. In 1982 more industrial action occurred than had taken place in either 1974 or in 1978/79. However, in 1983, in recognition of the fact that the RCN steadfastly maintained a 'no strike' policy, the Prime Minister established a pay review body for nurses, midwives and professional, technical and ancillary staff. With hindsight this was probably the highest point for nursing since the establishment of the NHS in 1948. Nurse administrators enjoyed a parity of influence with medical staff and administrators, the arrangements for determining their pay were on an equal footing with the medical and dental professions and were more favourable than those for administrative and clerical staff. As a consequence of the management arrangements introduced in 1972 (DHSS 1972), nursing was the one discipline that had a clear hierarchical relationship between staff providing direct patient care and the chief officer positions on district management teams. The managerial functionalism that the Grey Book arrangements encouraged had reinforced the strength of the nursing profession.

However, in February 1983 an event occurred which was to eliminate many of the perceived gains. Sir Roy Griffiths, the Deputy Chairman and Managing Director of Sainsbury's, was asked by Norman Fowler to undertake a management review of the NHS. The initial terms of reference were drawn up to focus on the utilization and management of manpower but at Sir Roy's request the terms of reference were drawn more widely. In October 1983 the NHS Management Inquiry Report was published in the form of a letter to the Secretary of State. The Griffiths Report (as it is widely known) proposed that general managers should be appointed throughout the NHS (DHSS 1983). Through the establishment of the principle of general management one person would be held accountable at each level, planning change, effecting its implementation and controlling resources. Thus the gains that the nursing profession had made through the implementation of the Salmon Report and through consensus management were all lost. Following the appointment of general managers throughout the service many district general managers either abolished the post of district nursing officer or so changed the nature of the role that the influence and standing of the nursing profession was felt by nurses to be badly affected.

Partly in response to the feeling of grievance amongst senior nurses, the RCN spent a quarter of a million pounds on a major advertising campaign against the proposals contained within the Griffiths Report. However, the government was determined to try to improve the management and control of resources within the service and to proceed with the proposal. There was also clear evidence that general managers in looking for savings (real or illusory) saw the nursing budget as a major target. Hence, whilst the 1970s and the early 1980s had seen a steady enhancement of the status of the nursing profession, the post-Griffiths period from 1984 onwards saw the reverse. In effecting these changes many general managers had the willing support of those consultants who had always felt that the only useful nurse was a bedside nurse, and that the Salmon Report was a piece of misguided nonsense exceeded only in the damage it inflicted on the service by the management structures imposed on them by the recommendations of the Grey Book.

It must be a matter of concern that the standing and the morale of many of those who were responsible for managing nursing services was adversely affected at a time when it was going to be increasingly difficult to recruit new entrants to the nursing and midwifery professions. Yet the sustained effect of RAWP on health authorities in London and other large urban centres, such as

Birmingham, the continued underfunding of pay, price inflation and the pressure being exerted on the service to be more productive and to exercise better financial control, placed many health authorities in an extremely difficult position. The elimination of effective nursing leadership in many DHAs must have had an effect on staff morale and the degree to which the many nurses providing direct patient care felt supported and encouraged by leaders from their own profession.

In the autumn of 1987 the financial problems facing many health authorities became a matter of public concern, most of the early publicity focusing on the shortage of nursing staff in the intensive care unit at the Birmingham Children's Hospital. The publication in January 1989 of the White Paper *Working for Patients* (DoH *et al.* 1989b) and the consequences of its subsequent enactment promises to introduce to the NHS some of the economic rigours that the commercial sector of the UK economy faced between 1979 and 1983. Yet the proposals also contain advantages that are as available to the nursing profession as to any other group of staff. The separation of the purchaser role in new DHAs from that of the provider of health services presents the opportunity for a much more explicit analysis of the health needs of the population and the setting of service specifications to meet those needs. Accompanying the analysis of need must be a rigorous assessment and evaluation of the most effective and most economic ways of meeting those needs.

One major consequence arising from the implementation of *Working for Patients* will be that national grading structures and, increasingly, national pay determination mechanisms will cease to have relevance. The way care is organized, the way it is provided for patients, and the way in which resources are used in the provision of that care are going to be the subject of continuous, detailed scrutiny and review. Whilst many nurses may regret the passing significance of the Pay Review Body, the Nurses and Midwives Whitley Council, and the general process of regulation of the grading structures and remuneration at national level, in those authorities and self-governing trusts where effective management provides the necessary leadership and skills to deliver the White Paper changes, then all staff, including nurses, should find their jobs though demanding, more satisfying. Moreover, as individuals they will share in the economic gains arising from a more productive use of resources. The relationship between organizational success and personal reward will be strengthened as never before. This will require rigour from the nursing profession in analysing those skills and associated training that are required to provide good quality care to patients. Increasingly, the unsatisfactory position of unqualified nursing staff being left in charge of acutely ill patients, especially at night, and other manifestations of a poor quality service, must disappear. Those self-governing trusts or directly managed units that fail to provide good quality services to patients will be penalized heavily.

Moreover, the government may find that a greater proportion of the gross domestic product has to be spent on health care in order to meet quality standards. However, I do anticipate that, during the first seven years following the enactment of the recommendations of the White Paper *Working for Patients*, substantial productivity gains will be realized within the NHS as pressure is put on clinicians, in particular, to change clinical practice. The considerable freedom that many clinicians have enjoyed in organizing their working life as they see fit will come under closer scrutiny. Within these reforms there are two significant opportunities for nurses. First, those who enjoy improving their clinical knowledge and expertise will have an opportunity to expand their area of work and take on tasks that have traditionally been undertaken by medical staff. Second, those nurses who genuinely enjoy a general management role will have an opportunity to exercise their skills and authority in continually reviewing the way that resources are deployed to give care to patients. Their remit will extend much more widely than nursing. The members of the nursing profession who have seen their role primarily as an administrative one, acting in a consensus and representational mode, will find the new requirement impossible to meet. Thus for some members of the profession – and this applies to all disciplines in the health service – this most recent reform represents either a tremendous opportunity or an appalling threat. One thing is clear, there will not be much ground between those options.

Looking positively, some work has already been undertaken in many DHAs in the form of skill mix reviews. However, the fundamental multi-disciplinary appraisal of the efficacy of care and the best way of organizing resources to provide that care for patients will in future be much more rigorous and all embracing. Nurses will not only have to extend their clinical skills but also acquire a much wider range of managerial skills than they have had to hitherto. Some of the tensions that were evident when the clinical nurse grading structure was introduced in the autumn of 1987 will resurface. Issues of competence, responsibility and skills will not be able to be fudged in the way they have in the past. Whilst this change will cause some unhappiness it is a process that will need to be borne. The link between skills, productivity and personal reward will become explicit.

This cultural change is being introduced at a time when labour market conditions are particularly disadvantageous to the NHS. Much has been written elsewhere about the decline in the number of school leavers in the population and the consequences of this for recruitment to the nursing profession. However, from a national economic perspective the resolution of this problem may not give rise to gloom. The wastage rate from many schools of nursing is a disgrace and the attrition and turnover rates experienced in most health authorities are far too high. In addition, amongst the large number of qualified nurses in the community who are not currently working in health care there lies the potential for resolving the recruitment problems facing the service, should the NHS continue to require the same number of staff currently in post. For what cannot be ignored is that when other organizations in Britain which have hitherto been run as public sector corporations have experienced the economic and market-related pressures that the NHS is going to face as a result of the enactment of the White Paper, required levels of staffing have reduced significantly. I believe that at the end of this decade we may find that there has been a reduction, perhaps as high as 25 per cent, in the total labour force in the NHS and that some of that reduction will have occurred in the nursing profession. Just as nurses have been recruited wastefully, they have probably been deployed wastefully, and waste is something that no provider unit will be able to afford in the future.

The choice and its outcomes are clear. The successful implementation of the White Paper reforms may well lead to a smaller workforce working more flexibly, with a higher skill and knowledge base, working more productively and gaining higher personal rewards – and perhaps higher satisfaction as well.

The alternative is a stagnant labour force that does not increase its knowledge and skill base, continues to work within the context of national pay, conditions of service and grading structures, and displays the worst characteristics of a bureaucratic system by providing services of declining quality. Achieving the more positive outcome is not going to be easy but few people can be better placed to do so than the more able and enterprising nurses within the service. The question must be, are there enough of them and will they be given the support and leadership to sustain their choice?

5

Nurse and doctor: Whose task is it anyway?

Martin McKee and Leila Lessof

Nurses, it is often claimed, are no longer the handmaidens of doctors. In this chapter, Martin McKee and Leila Lessof examine the changing relationship between nursing and medicine, charting moves that have recently taken place to extend and expand the role of the nurse. The chapter raises some challenging issues. The authors ask whether opposition by some segments of the medical profession to nurses' enhanced role represents a concern about standards of patient care; or whether such opposition reflects a protectionist occupational stance, a desire to safeguard doctors' jobs. Further, the authors raise questions about whether the goal of simply carrying out technical tasks delegated by doctors is a goal which nursing ought to be striving towards. Martin McKee and Leila Lessof write, of course, from a medical perspective and some nurses would argue that extending their role to take on jobs that doctors might wish to delegate is of a different order to an expanded role. The latter is much more in line with the view of nursing responsibilities advanced by the proponents of the 'New Nursing'. Finally, through a fascinating look at events currently taking place in the USA, Martin McKee and Leila Lessof draw our attention to the kinds of conflict that may yet be experienced in this country.

Introduction

> It seems a commonly received idea among men, and even among women themselves, that it requires nothing but a disappointment in love, or incapacity in other things, to turn a woman into a good nurse.
>
> (Florence Nightingale in Woodham-Smith 1950: 340)

Traditionally nursing has been seen as an extension of the work women do in the home (Salvage 1990b), and nurses are viewed as a relatively unskilled, subordinate group of doctors' helpers. The dominance of the medical profession has been comprehensive with doctors having a key role in deciding what student nurses should be taught and, later, in nursing appointments (Mitchell 1984).

This doctor–nurse relationship was not all it seemed. In the 'doctor–nurse' game, as described by Stein in 1967, the doctor was deemed to be superior to the nurse and to make all important treatment decisions, but in practice many of the decisions were suggested by the nurse. However, the idea of the game was that it appeared that the doctor had thought of them first. The game suited all sides and ensured a co-operative and efficient working relationship. However, there have been considerable changes in both medicine and nursing since Stein's original article (Stein *et al.* 1990).

The role of women in society is changing and the proportion of female medical graduates and independent 'therapy' professionals has risen. The therapists have made it abundantly clear that they are autonomous professionals and are not subordinate to doctors. This has disrupted the rules of the game which were derived largely from a gender-based hierarchy. The technical expertise of the nurse has expanded in parallel with the increasing complexity of modern medicine, especially in areas such as intensive and neonatal care, nephrology and cardiology. Nurses are working as equals in inter-disciplinary teams in psychiatry and geriatric medicine. Finally, some nurses are acting as independent practitioners in certain specialist posts and in occupational health.

The desire among nurses for increased professionalism and greater autonomy is now apparent. Nurses increasingly view themselves as health-care professionals with equal status to doctors (Delamothe 1988). The reform of nurse education, as embodied in Project 2000, will provide a more academic basis in training and will provide for a specialist practitioner grade (UKCC 1986a). The Cumberlege Report (DHSS 1986a) has advocated the establishment of nurse practitioners in the community.

Changes in medicine

Changes in medicine have led some doctors to welcome the extended role of the nurse, notably in the context of the delegation of technical tasks. Because of an increasing concern about the excessive hours worked by junior doctors (*The Times* 1988: 3), several studies have demonstrated how many of the night tasks for which junior doctors are called could be equally well done by the nurse who calls them (DHSS 1971; Astill and Watkin 1987; Upton 1989). There are, however, bureaucratic obstacles to prevent this happening and an experienced staff nurse may find herself calling a newly qualified house officer to the ward at night in order to explain exactly what needs to be done, or even a more senior doctor who has not previously performed a technically complex procedure, such as the insertion of a pace-maker. Patient care may suffer when an intravenous drug is given several hours late because the house-officer was busy elsewhere, while in a neighbouring hospital the drug would be given on time during the nurse's drug round.

The suggestion that nurses should assume a larger role in patient care is echoed by working groups which have examined this issue. If the long hours worked by junior doctors are to be reduced, leading to fewer mistakes and safer treatment, it may be necessary for nurses to assume responsibility for many of these tasks (*Nursing Standard* 1988).

This is already happening in some areas. Changes in hospital medical staffing in the 1990s will lead to a considerable reduction in the number of registrars (DHSS 1986b). In a few obstetric units this has already happened, and mid-wives have successfully taken over many of the areas of responsibility under-taken by doctors (Green *et al.* 1986).

Despite the considerable pressure for an enhanced role for nursing, progress has been slow and there has been a wide variation among hospitals in the extent to which nurses have extended their role. The possible reasons for this include perceived official barriers and ingrained professional attitudes. These will be examined in turn.

Do rules constrain the extension of the role of nursing?

The role of the nurse is governed by the Nurses, Midwives and Health Visitors Act (1979) which does not contain restrictions on the tasks that a nurse may carry out. The Briggs Committee (Briggs 1972) recognized that the traditional differences in some of the functions of doctors and nurses were becoming less distinguishable and also noted the absence of legal constraints on what might be undertaken by nurses. The Committee proposed, however, that nurses should only perform those duties for which they have received training and this was translated into policy in Health Circular HC(77)22 (DHSS 1977). As a result, health authorities were asked to review areas of clinical activity in which delegation to nurses would be desirable. The tone of the circular nevertheless supported a dominant role for medicine, using terms such as delegation and stressing the need for a clearly defined policy agreed with doctors.

The scope for delegation appears to be considerable if local agreement can be achieved. Tasks can be delegated if the nurse concerned is specifically trained and agrees to accept it, and if the training is accepted as satisfactory by the employing authority. New tasks should be recognized by both the employing authority and the professions as appropriate to be delegated, and the delegating doctor should be assured of the competence of the nurse.

The major professional organizations have accepted the principle of an extended nursing role, and the BMA and the RCN have stated that tasks which should be considered as extended clinical duties are 'those duties allocated to nurses which appear to be outside the generally accepted and current scope of nursing practice' (RCN/BMA 1978). The devolution of decision-making about an extended role for nurses to individual health authorities has contributed to the extensive variation in practice between and within hospitals. In hospitals where committees have developed policies they have often been designed *de novo*, without reference to the experience gained elsewhere.

The issue, more than any other, that has prevented individual nurses adopting a more extended role is the requirement that each employing authority should recognize that training has been satisfactory. In practice this means that most health authorities will only accept a certificate of competence if they have issued it themselves. Thus, while it may be agreed that nurses can give intravenous injections in a hospital, it may be that only a small number can actually do so and that even certificates issued within the same district may be queried. This is a particular problem in hospitals with a high staff turnover and large numbers of agency staff.

While legislation relating to nursing does not specifically limit the role of the nurse, prescribing is an important area which is protected on behalf of anyone but a medical practitioner or, in certain circumstances, a dentist or veterinary surgeon. However, the role of the nurse in prescribing is beginning to be reconsidered. Existing legislation embodied in the Medicines Act (1968) precludes a nurse from administering a prescription-only drug except under the direction of a doctor. The relevant section of the Medicines Act states that:

> no person shall administer (otherwise than to himself) any such medicinal product unless he is an appropriate practitioner or a person acting in accordance with the directions of an appropriate practitioner.
>
> (Medicines Act 1968 para. 58:2:b)

It is permitted for a nurse to vary a dose of a drug or administer one in the absence of a prescription, but only within a specific set of locally negotiated guidelines. The relevant guidance is contained in an advisory paper from the UKCC which aims to assist the development of local policies (UKCC 1986b). While it identifies prescribing as the doctor's role it states that:

Instruction by telephone to a nurse to administer, even in an emergency situation, a hitherto unprescribed drug cannot be supported [although] Where it is the wish of the doctors that nursing staff be authorised to administer certain medicines such as mild analgesics, laxatives and topical applications a local protocol . . . should be agreed between the medical, nursing and pharmaceutical professionals involved.

(UKCC 1986b: paras 2g and 2h)

The UKCC recognizes that these recommendations are not absolute and that:

There are certain situations in which practitioners are involved in the administration of medicines where specific factors within the preceding framework are difficult to apply or could not be applied without introducing dangerous delay and its consequent risk to patients. These will include occupational nursing settings in industry, small hospitals with no resident medical staff and possibly some specialist units within larger hospitals and a variety of community settings.

(UKCC 1986b, supplement: 11)

It continues:

It is therefore recommended that, in any situation where practitioners might be called upon or expected to administer 'prescription only' medicines which have not been directly prescribed as a result of examination, the following principles should be agreed and set down in local policy which is known to all practitioners likely to be involved.
(i) It should first be agreed and then set down in writing by all the doctors working within that particular setting that there are circumstances in which particular 'prescription only' medicines may be administered in advance of examination by a doctor. Where frequent staff changes make this impractical one senior doctor should be appointed by his/her colleagues to establish such policies on their behalf, with them undertaking to honour his/her decision. A review of such policies must take place annually.
(ii) The particular circumstances in which a particular 'prescription only' medicine (and its form, route, etc.) could be administered must then be the subject of specific and well documented agreement which must have similar support.

(UKCC 1986b, supplement: 11)

The guidance also advises that nurses should only be able to act as above if they have undergone a specific course of instruction and have a written authority to administer a specific drug in a particular set of circumstances.

In the new circumstances that now obtain the constraints on nurse prescribing may be about to change, and it has now been suggested that prescribing by nurses should be permitted in certain circumstances. An advisory committee set up by the DoH has recommended amending the Medicines Act 1968 so that nurses should be able to prescribe (DoH 1989c). The effect of this would be that a nurse could refer to a nurses' formulary and prescribe certain items for conditions for which the nurse takes clinical responsibility, following a group protocol agreed for a particular clinical service. This would clearly represent a major expansion into what has traditionally been seen to be a medical responsibility. There will almost inevitably be pressure for a similar policy in hospitals, and this may be particularly appropriate for long-stay units. The Hospital Junior Staff Committee of the BMA has already suggested such a change (Beecham 1990).

Do nurses want to take over this role?

Two differing views of the role of nursing have been stereotyped as the 'caring' and 'curing' approaches (Salvage 1985: 5). The 'curing' group are anxious to expand their role to include more technical tasks. The 'caring' role is encapsulated by the definition of nursing as:

> assisting the patient to perform activities leading to better health, or a peaceful death, that he or she would normally perform unaided, given the strength, will, and knowledge.
>
> (Henderson 1966)

Those advocating the latter caring role have emphasized the need to develop technical skills within the context of nursing and to avoid being seen as a doctor's 'handmaiden' and attending to those jobs with which the doctors have become bored. As an example, there was widespread opposition from nursing organizations to the establishment of a post in which a nurse would dissect veins prior to cardiac surgery (*Nursing Standard* 1989). This is by no means a unanimous view, and there are many nurses, especially in the more technologically advanced areas of clinical practice, who would greet such posts with enthusiasm.

How will the medical profession respond to changes in nursing?

One of the major concerns voiced by doctors about an extended role for nurses concerns the adequacy of training. This is illustrated by the statement from a doctor that:

> no nurse is allowed to assume such an extended technical role without adequate training plus a certificate of competence from medical staff who are prepared to delegate such tasks to her.
>
> (Mitchell 1984)

This view is supported by HC(77)22 (DHSS 1977) which requires specific additional training which must be recognized by all concerned. This is in striking contrast to the situation for doctors. Once doctors qualify there is an implicit assumption that they are skilled in all of the tasks necessary for the diagnosis and treatment of patients under their care or that, if they are not, they will call for assistance as required. With nurses it is assumed that the skill is absent unless it has been taught and tested.

The assumption that newly qualified doctors possess skills which are denied to nurses is hard to justify. It is only in recent times that the need to provide specific training for medical students in cardiac resuscitation has been recognized (Skinner 1985) and this training is often provided by nurses (G. Wynne, unpublished observations). It has even been alleged that only one medical school in the United Kingdom teaches medical students how to give intravenous drugs (Bain *et al.* 1990).

Although some doctors have expressed concern about the adequacy of training for those nurses who may take on an extended role, the medical profession in the UK seems to favour the idea of nurses performing more clinical activities in hospital. Reservations about an extended role are, however, beginning to emerge in the community health services, and the Central Consultants and Specialists Committee have considered the proposals for nurse prescribing and expressed concern about them (Beecham 1990).

It is difficult to judge how much of the concern expressed by the medical profession relates to the maintenance of standards and how much relates to a protectionist attitude and a concern about doctors' employment opportunities. Community health doctors have expressed their anxiety that health authorities may replace them with less expensive nurses (Merry 1990), and the ambivalent, paradoxical views which are held have been neatly illustrated in a letter to *Hospital Doctor* which drew attention to two juxtaposed articles in an earlier issue. One advocated that many routine tasks should be undertaken by nurse practitioners, while the other reported further developments in the long running campaign by the BMA to oppose the holding of blood transfusion sessions without doctors being present (Henderson 1990).

The perception of a threat to medicine from nursing has been much greater in the USA. Doctors there have felt increasingly threatened by the enhanced role and correspondingly improved status of nurses (Iglehart 1987). In particular they have been worried about proposals that would authorize the Health Care Financing Administration to contract with nursing service organizations for patient care on a pre-paid capitation basis. This may not reflect upon nursing competence, however, in a situation in which matters of finance appear to have received greater emphasis than standards of health care. The medical establishment in the USA has fought back on a number of fronts (Iglehart 1987). The American Medical Association (AMA) has withdrawn from a scheme to improve the educational and political status of nurses on the grounds that it is against the best interests of medicine. It is not clear whether the argument is based on the effectiveness of patient care or the relative status of physicians and nurses. It has been claimed that the American Society of Anesthesiologists has mounted a sustained campaign to eliminate the role of nurse-anaesthetists and the AMA has countered the expanded role of nursing by developing a new style of worker – the registered care technician (AMA 1989). These individuals would be accountable to doctors and principally responsible for carrying out their orders. Not surprisingly, nurses have opposed this development, seeing it as a means of recreating a group of subservient, low-status workers who will be dominated by physicians (O'Conner 1988).

The roles of doctors and nurses in the UK are changing. The challenge for both professions is to work together to avoid the conflicts that have occurred on the other side of the Atlantic so that the changes do not merely benefit both groups but also serve the ultimate purpose of improving care for the patient. The relationship of nurses to other health care professionals will also need consideration, as will the legal implications of their extended role – such as those related to drugs – which are not inconsiderable (DHSS 1977; DoH 1989c).

The future pattern of health care will also be affected, perhaps very substantially. Health services as they exist today mainly reflect the professional interests and concerns of the medical profession. The new arrangements envisage a greater influence for the professional interests and concerns of the nurse. Project 2000 (UKCC 1986a; 1987) notes that in training programmes for nurses, midwives' and health visitors' 'perceived service needs and perceived training needs can . . . come into conflict'. It is recommended on educational grounds and to slow the drift of nurses away from the profession that the nursing student should be supernumerary to NHS staffing establishments and no longer included in duty rotas. While it is assumed that nursing aides or support workers can fill the students nurses' caring role, it is by no means clear that this plan can fulfil the overall needs of the service. To some extent the managerial changes following from the White Paper *Working for Patients* (DoH *et al.* 1989b) may, however, help to keep the needs of training and health care in balance, by allowing DHAs to purchase the services that they believe will best meet the needs of their resident populations. This will offer a great deal of scope for new types and patterns of service development. Undoubtedly, there will be a need for negotiation, but there will also be major opportunities for the extended role of the nurse acting as an independent and autonomous practitioner.

It will be interesting to see how the medical profession responds. An unsigned editorial in the *Lancet* (1990) recently re-stated the issues involved in any reappraisal of the roles of doctor and nurse. The letters written in response, whether supporting a traditional approach or advocating reform, show clearly that this is still a burning issue arousing strong emotions.

6

Nursing policy and the nationalization of nursing: The representation of 'crisis' and the 'crisis' of representation

Anne Marie Rafferty

In this chapter, Anne Marie Rafferty explores the notion of a 'crisis' in nursing through an historical perspective. Focusing on the problems of recruitment and retention experienced during the inter-war years, Anne Marie Rafferty illustrates her contention that it is only through the transformation of nursing issues into 'crises' that such issues reach the public agenda. But whilst nursing issues may reach the public policy agenda, nurses themselves have played little part in either setting the agenda or in the process of formulating policy. Drawing on historical evidence from the period immediately before and during the early NHS, Anne Marie Rafferty documents how poorly nursing interests were represented in the policy arena, with nurses themselves playing only a very limited role in the policy-making process. Questions concerning nursing policy, Anne Marie Rafferty argues, have always been subsumed by health service planners under wider questions concerning the health service in general, in the expectation that nurses will simply conform to whatever role is imposed upon them. Anne Marie Rafferty concludes by drawing attention to what she characterizes as a 'crisis in confidence' in nursing.

Introduction

This chapter addresses the assumption of a crisis in nursing from the perspective of historical policy-analysis. First the meaning of 'crisis' is explored with reference to recruitment difficulties during the inter-war period. It is argued that the definition of 'crisis' requires contextualization and that historical research provides a useful analytic tool for exploring its different dimensions and applications. Nursing policy is considered in terms of the participation of nurses in central advisory and policy-making machinery before and during the early NHS. It is argued that nurses sought access to policy-making bodies as a precursor to setting their own agenda for change. The case for nurses attempting to set their own policy agenda receives only weak support from the evidence considered here. It is argued that the origin and 'career' of policy decisions related to nursing are best understood in the context of their relationship to wider health care policy concerns and governmental objectives.

The evidence presented in this chapter lends some support for the assumption that it is primarily in terms of 'crisis' that nursing issues reach the public policy agenda. Whilst labour shortages may be important triggers for focusing attention upon problems in the nursing services, they are not in themselves sufficient to ensure that action and measurable policy outcomes will follow. They may temporarily destabilize political and economic systems without fundamentally altering the character of those institutions. In this sense they may resemble what Held refers to as a partial crisis in which a phase of temporary stability is interrupted rather than a crisis of 'transformative potential' which challenges the very core of the political and social order (Held 1989). A combination of several pressures, and escalating anxieties which threaten public confidence in health care are more likely to stimulate a more serious response from the stakeholders of power. The 'crises' that have occurred in nursing seem to be lacking in what Held calls 'transformational potential'. Negotiating the meaning of 'crisis' may be one of the major tasks confronting policy-makers engaged in reconciling conflicting interests of competing groups. In the sections that follow I shall explore the extent to which nurses as one of many competing interest groups, succeeded in setting their own policy-agenda in the early NHS.

The meaning of crisis

The medical and dramaturgical meaning of 'crisis' is one of a turning point and this may connote a change for the better or worse. In contemporary usage it conveys the sense of difficulty, insecurity or suspense in politics or commerce (*Oxford English Dictionary*). 'Crises' in nursing derive from a range of perceived sources. They may be epidemiological, demographic, economic, or as with the AIDS epidemic, a combination of all three. Definitions of what constitutes a crisis varies according to context, and meanings are not self-evident but require witnesses and political actors to give expression to them. In this sense they can be considered constructions whose urgency is often conveyed by apocalyptic language. Labour 'shortages' in nursing are often represented as 'crises' and give rise to gloomy prognostications encapsulated within such phrases as 'demographic timebomb'. To illustrate the vagaries of 'diagnosing' and 'treating' manpower 'crises' in nursing I shall review the career of such a 'crisis' in the inter-war period.

Nursing shortages

Before the establishment of the NHS no routine statistics were collected on the employment of nurses and no authority had overall responsibility for monitoring manpower levels. The only statistical record submitted to the MoH on a regular basis was the annual return of new registrations from the General Nursing Council (GNC) for England and Wales (MoH 1920–39). Assessment of nursing 'shortages' during the inter-war period were made through combining professional judgement and statistical evidence derived from numbers of unfilled vacancies collected by hospitals. Both methods were used by the Lancet Commission which it supplemented by its own independent survey conducted by the statistician and epidemiologist Austin (later Sir) Bradford Hill (*Lancet* 1931a, b: 1932).

The symptoms of crisis in nursing manpower in sanatoria

The alarm about the impending nursing manpower crisis was first raised by Dr Esther Carling, medical superintendent of a sanatorium in 1930 (Carling 1930). As one of the least popular, prestigious and most depressed areas of nursing work, tuberculosis nursing can be considered a barometer of the climatic changes in the nursing labour market. Dr Carling's letter was published in the *Lancet* which, in keeping with its campaigning tradition of the nineteenth century, launched a Commission to inquire into the reasons behind the shortage. Its findings revealed a qualitative and quantitative shortfall in recruitment and retention of 'educated' candidates. The principal cause was diagnosed as chronic neglect of conditions of service and outmoded attitudes: nursing had failed to modernize and as a consequence was losing any previous competitive advantage over supposedly rival occupations such as social work and business (Robinson and Rafferty 1988: 52). The assumption underlying these assertions was that nursing had previously not only competed favourably for secondary educated recruits but that middle-class social and educational backgrounds were characteristic of recruits to nursing. This latter assumption was contradicted by evidence submitted to the Commission which stated that some hospitals had to be content 'so long as candidates could read and write' (*Lancet*

1931b: v). Moreover a memorandum to the Commission from the Education Committee of the County of Worcester in June 1931 stated that only six out of 740 secondary school leavers had taken up nursing (Robinson and Rafferty 1988: 53).

From crisis to complacency

Although the Lancet Commission proved useful as a consciousness-raising exercise, it produced few tangible improvements in recruitment or conditions. The deficiencies it exposed provided ample ammunition for reformers to petition employing authorities to institute improvements but no such opportunity was seized. Instead it was superseded by changes in labour market conditions which allowed employers to lapse into a *laissez-faire* mode of operation. In 1933, only one year after the panic about manpower shortages had been publicized, the *Lancet* too seemed sanguine: 'the express purpose of attracting candidates for training has during the past year become less urgent, because the influx of suitable young women into the nursing profession has greatly increased' (*Lancet* 1933: 369). The deteriorating economic climate was perceived as responsible for the upturn in recruitment 'during which any form of training offering board and lodging and pocket money has advantages' (p. 369). Indeed the temporary improvement in recruitment was considered sufficiently threatening for the RCN to advance a protectionist employment policy against the admission of foreign probationers to British Hospitals for training (MoH 1933). This turn-around from crisis to complacency in nurse recruitment provides an illustration of the extent to which the term 'crisis' requires contextual interpretation.

The cycle of events

The reluctance of the College of Nursing to petition and pressurize relevant agencies into taking decisive action to improve conditions of service and, in particular, to rationalize superannuation anomalies diminished in the mid-1930s. The College lobbied the MoH from 1935 onwards to establish national pay negotiation machinery jointly with National Association of Local Government Offices (NALGO) but was keen to distance itself from Trade Union Congress (TUC) affiliated trade unions. Independent investigations commissioned by the College had revealed the extent of poor conditions of service in the different branches of the occupation. In spite of this awareness the College was defensive in the face of criticisms regarding conditions of service which originated from sources other than itself. These were interpreted as an oblique charge that the College had failed to secure improvements themselves. Criticisms appearing in the national press were a particular source of embarrassment (*Daily Express* 1937, *Daily Sketch* 1937a, *Nottingham Journal and Express*

1937). Nurses found they had many champions ready to support their cause including such public figures as the actress Sybil Thorndike (*Daily Sketch* 1937b). Support from popular figures and celebrities arguably added to the weight of public opinion sympathetic to nurses' well publicized plight. A deluge of criticism on nursing conditions appeared in the national press between 1936 and 1937, projecting nursing issues onto the public policy arena.

Although the short-term problem of labour shortage subsided in the mid-1930s, this was achieved mainly by substituting assistant for student nurses. The relief was transient and the twin pressures of economic recession combined with increasing demand for labour renewed anxieties of 'crisis'. Furthermore the practice of labour substitution stimulated a wave of unionization by nurses. The TUC pressed for modernization of working conditions through its sponsorship of a Nurses' Charter and resuscitated attempts to introduce employment legislation in the form of a Limitation of Hours Bill (TUC 1937).

Sensing the threat of union rivalry, the College of Nursing forged an alliance with the non-TUC affiliated NALGO to establish joint national negotiating machinery for pay and conditions in the hope of recapturing some of the political territory lost to the unions. This proposal was put to the MoH along with a request for an inquiry into the supply and demand for trained nurses in the community in 1935. Both requests came to nought. In 1937 the College reiterated its request for a government inquiry, capitalizing upon the combined pressures of industrial militancy and parliamentary lobbying for a policy response to the TUC's Limitation of Hours Bill. These pressures supplemented with well-documented grievances of nurses in the press, were sufficient to induce the government to set up a Committee of Inquiry in order to buy time in the hope that the situation would stabilize.

The Inter-Departmental Committee on Nursing Services (which later became known as the Athlone Committee) was established in 1937 as a governmental response to the culminating pressures (MoH, Board of Education 1939). The Committee was asked to inquire into arrangements currently operating in relation to recruitment, training and conditions of service and recommend changes necessary to maintain an adequate institutional or domiciliary nursing service. The Committee worked quickly and produced an interim report in 1939. The wartime emergency had contradictory implications for government intervention in nursing; it provided a temporary excuse for government inaction on the Committee's findings but at the same time necessitated a more rational approach to the planning and formulation of policy in the nursing services (Dingwall *et al.* 1988: 103).

Representational policy

The meaning of policy is not self-evident and different commentators have stressed different aspects of its constitution. Considerable debate surrounds the question of whether policy is more than an intended course of action, whether it includes the behaviour involved in implementing that action as well as the outcome of implementation whether intended or not (Heclo 1972). As an analytic category 'policy' like 'crisis' can be most clearly defined with reference to empirical evidence. Uncovering the intentions, declared or ascribed, of policy-makers requires detailed qualitative analysis of the nuances of decision-making. Such refined detail is rarely contained in documentary sources and is best extracted from oral accounts. The present discussion draws upon documentary rather than oral or interview sources and focuses on how nurses gained representation on policy-making bodies rather than the determinants and determination of policy-making itself. Representation has to do with making something present which was previously absent (Pitkin 1967). The task of policy-makers in nursing therefore might be construed as making nursing visible where it might otherwise be invisible.

Nurse representation on national bodies

The articulation of deep dissatisfaction with the representational role of nurses in policy-making and decision-making is not of recent origin although translating such protest into a national campaign most certainly is (Owen and Glennister 1990; Strong and Robinson 1990: 27). A series of abortive attempts were made by nurses to gain representation on government health-policy-advisory machinery between 1919 and 1939 (Rafferty 1988). Yet in the end it was not on the basis of demand from the nursing organizations but necessity borne of the needs of wartime planning that nurses were eventually included in central health policy-making machinery.

When the Second World War commenced there was only a handful of nurses on the staff of the MoH and none had the experience of recruiting and directing large numbers of nurses necessary to meet the needs of the Emergency Medical Services (EMS). Some had previously been employed as Women Inspectors of Poor Law Hospitals and Maternal and Child Welfare Services. They had not, however, been employed to offer nursing advice to policy-makers. Planning for the needs of the EMS had an inevitable impact on nursing. The main short-term problem for nursing was providing an adequate service to civilians and the military within a system of increasing but fluctuating demands. Throughout the course of the war, the government assumed increasing financial responsibility for the nursing services. National bargaining machinery for the determination of salaries and conditions of service was established in 1941 under Lord Rushcliffe who produced a first report in 1943 recommending substantial increases to female staff (MoH *et al.* 1943). The report was rapidly accepted and implemented but had a limited effect on the supply of nurses. The Committee's approach actually intensified the problems of distribution. Nurses and hospitals colluded to evade attempts to direct staff where they were thought to be most needed (especially to tuberculosis sanatoria, hospitals for the chronically ill, mentally ill and maternity cases). Furthermore national pay scales had abolished the pay differentials that formerly had been an aid to recruitment in unpopular specialisms.

It was only to a limited extent that the Nursing Division of the MoH, established in 1941, could influence the distribution of labour. Miss Katherine Watt, recently retired from the post of air-commandant of Princess Mary's Royal Air Force Nursing Service had taken over the task of nurse deployment in 1939, in which she was supported by Gladys Fletcher, Secretary of the London branch of the RCN. Miss Watt became the first Chief Nursing Officer (CNO) at the Ministry in 1941. She then had two deputies to help her in addition to Miss Fletcher, one for Public Health the other for the Hospital Services. This number later increased to twenty-one women inspectors and twenty-three regional Nursing Officers responsible for allocating posts to members of the Civil Nursing Reserve (women with previous training and experience and untrained volunteers/nursing 'auxiliaries') from the Headquarters of the Regional Offices and maintaining an even distribution of nurses to the hospitals in the regions (Cockayne 1988).

The problem of nurse deployment was only alleviated to any degree when the Control of Engagement order covering women aged 18–40 years was applied to nursing in September 1943. In effect this meant the conscription of nurses. Unless they were undertaking further training, nurses could only leave their current appointment for one on a priority list maintained by the Ministry of Labour. This loophole exempting those undertaking further training was widely exploited in order to evade the regulations. It led on the one hand to the benefit of maternity hospitals offering midwifery courses but, on the other, to the continuing detriment of other shortage areas (Webster 1985). Eventually in April 1944, the Ministry took the power to direct newly qualified nurses away from their training schools to relieve shortages elsewhere. The 'further training' exemption remained, however, with the result that 91 per cent of newly qualified nurses elected to go onto other courses rather than allowing their employment to be directed by the Ministry (Dingwall *et al.* 1988).

The Ministry of Labour and National Service (MLNS), as the major department responsible for the recruitment and deployment of manpower, established a National Advisory Council for the Recruitment and Distribution of Nurses and Midwives in 1941. Shared responsibility for the recruitment and deployment of Nurses and Midwives, however, generated tension and territorial disputes between the two Ministries. The MLNS maintained responsibility for organizing recruitment campaigns, monitoring staff vacancies and even placing students until 1957 when its functions were transferred to the MoH (MLNS 1957).

The nationalization of nursing

The experience of wartime health services had two important consequences for nursing. One was the acceptance by all political parties that there could not be a return to the pre-war heterogeneity of health care provision. Many of the emergency arrangements were destined to become permanent institutions in the post-welfare state. As a result nursing would take its place within a more uniform framework of planning and administration. The formation of the NHS has been discussed in detail elsewhere (Webster 1988). The key point here, however, is just how much of the previous structure was left intact. The only genuine administrative innovations came in the hospital sector with the merging of voluntary and municipal hospitals. Three tiers of administration were constructed: below the Ministry came fourteen Regional Hospital Boards (RHBs) and 377 Hospital Management Committees (HMCs), in England and Wales. But the picture was complicated by concessions to traditional interests. As part of the Ministry's strategy for overcoming BMA opposition, thirty-six teaching hospitals were given independent status, with their own Boards of Governors reporting directly to the Minister. Throughout the drafting of NHS legislation there was remarkably little evidence of pressure from nursing organizations for consultation on this or indeed any other aspect of early NHS policy.

The absence of a nursing lobby was referred to by Mrs Blair-Fish, an officer of the RCN in a speech at the annual professional conference of the College in December 1944 on the Future Health Services. She expressed the College's disappointment that the then Minister of Health, Mr Harry Willink, guest speaker at the conference, had not consulted the nursing profession as he had the medical profession during early negotiations. 'Perhaps nurses were to blame' she added 'they knew the plans were brewing and had their hands not been so full they could have collected a statement from College members and stormed the steps of Whitehall, but the opportunity was lost' (*Nursing Times* 1944: 844). The hints outlined in the White Paper that nurses should take part in the planning of the new services and should have representation on the national and local advisory councils, were welcomed by the College Council. The fear that nurses might not have full rights of participation in the new structure was expressed: 'if nursing were only dealt with by a sub-committee', it was stated, 'the Minister would find the baby too big for the pram' (p. 845). Mr Willink reassured conference delegates that nurses would be represented on advisory machinery at national, and local levels as well as having their own sub-committee within central advisory machinery (p. 845).

The central advisory machinery

Two things are striking about the history of nursing policy in the early health service: the first is the very limited participation of nurses in the determination of nursing policy and the second is the inseparability of nursing from the wider concerns of health care planning. Nursing representatives selected for positions on governmental advisory machinery were generally elected through relevant sub-committees of the nursing organizations. The RCN had been perceived by the MoH as the chief source of advice on routine 'professional' or technical matters. The participation and opinion of trade unions was reserved more for specialized advice on employment or manpower issues although the government was careful to ensure their inclusion in committees likely to attract public attention.

At national level there was an elaborate professional advisory machinery which did conform to a more standard pattern. The 1946 NHS Act provided for a Central Health Services Council (CHSC) which set up a number of specialist Standing Advisory Committees (SACs). Nursing was the subject of one, maternity and midwifery another and mental health including mental nursing a third. The Standing Nursing Advisory Committee for Nursing (SNAC) had a narrow majority of nurse members in 1949. It is difficult to assess the impact of the SNAC upon Ministry policy but it was certainly one of the more active committees with a regular programme of quarterly meetings. In the first decade of its existence it dealt with a wide range of topics ranging from nursing techniques to cross-infection, the selection of nurse recruits and the sensitive issue of the employment of juveniles in hospitals. A number of other issues proved divisive, including the secondment of student nurses to TB sanatoria, to relieve the continued chronic staff shortages, and the use of enrolled nurses in mental and mental deficiency hospitals. A number of the SNACs recommendations were implemented as policy such as the establish-ment of the Joint Board of Clinical Nursing Studies (JBCNS) in 1972 to regulate the provision of post-certificate clinical training for nurses, an initiative that originated from a SNAC sub-committee report published in 1966 (CHSC 1966). This should not be seen solely as a victory for SNAC, however, as the first request for regulation of post-certificate clinical nursing courses had emanated from the GNC in 1943. Successive governments thus managed to postpone formal accreditation of post-registration clinical courses for nurses for thirty years before regulatory machinery was set up and it is only recently that demands for financial recognition of these qualifications are being dealt with.

Nursing Division within the Ministry of Health

In addition to the central advisory committees, the MoH also had a small Nursing Division, created during the war to oversee the direction of labour. This was staffed by administrative civil servants advised initially by a central group of five professional Nursing Officers who were on the miscellaneous staff of the Chief Medical Officer (CMO). Slowly the numbers and range of duties performed by Nursing Division developed until by 1964 it consisted of twenty-five Nursing Officers (NOs) working under a Chief Nursing Officer (CNO).

The Division had a central supervisory rather than executive role and its main task was to give professional advice on matters of policy affecting all aspects of the nursing services and nursing education including nursing administration, planning equipment, recruitment and manpower, basic, post-basic and in-service education. In terms of size the Nursing Division was considerably smaller than the Medical Division which employed eighty as opposed to twenty-six officers, and the CNO lacked parity with the CMO who reported directly to the Minister. The CNO attended all major meetings of the Whitley Council, CHSC, SNAC, RHB executive meetings, senior administrative medical officers' meetings and those of the chairmen of the RHBs. Contact was maintained with the regions via Regional Nursing Officers (RNOs) who liaised with RHBs and some NOs had specialist responsibilities for services such as mental and public health nursing and latterly nursing research. It is difficult to assess the impact of the Nursing Division upon departmental thinking, but as a supervisory rather than executive body, the Division's effectiveness may have depended more on the extent to which the CNO could influence the major committees of which she was a member than on her position within the DoH service.

Service issues

The 1944 White Paper (MoH 1944) did not specify the constitution of either RHBs or HMCs beyond providing that the Ministry should consult local universities involved in medical training, local authorities and such bodies as he thought appropriate. In fact there was considerable opposition to appointing people in any sort of representative capacity. The TUC questioned this in 1946 and was firmly disabused by Bevan, Minister of Health, of any notion that representation would be made on a proportionate, symbolic or mandatory basis. In a letter to Sir Walter Citrine, the TUC's general secretary, Bevan argued:

> ... bodies shall consist of members appointed for individual suitability and experience, and not as representatives or delegates of particular, and possibly conflicting interests. This means that members of RHBs and HMCs could not be appointed to 'represent' the health workers. . . . The difficulty here would be to draw any line which would keep membership of the Boards and Committees down to reasonable numbers. If the nurses were to be consulted, why not the hospital domestics? The radiotherapists? The physiotherapists? And so on?
>
> (Bevan, cited in Klein 1983: 21)

When coupled with a desire to avoid any possible accusation of political bias in appointments, the result was a set of nominations which virtually eliminated any labour movement and nursing interests and produced a structure controlled by those formerly playing similar roles in the voluntary hospitals (Webster 1988). A handful of nurses were appointed to these new bodies. The RHBs included thirteen nurses but they dwindled to seven in 1956 and one in 1974. This may reflect the increasing difficulty of deflecting demands from other groups of workers for comparable representation (Webster 1988). By contrast the medical profession, whose goodwill was more eagerly sought and whose opposition set a high price for co-operation, obtained 29 per cent of the appointments in 1947 and increased this to 31 per cent in 1956 although there was considerable regional variation within this range (Webster 1988).

If nursing received scant attention at this level of administration little is known about its influence through local hospital management channels. There was great variation in the extent to which HMCs consulted matrons and delegated powers to their officers but further research is required before any general patterns can be established.

White maintains that the administrative changes brought about by the NHS significantly undermined the power and authority of matrons (White 1986b). She argued that the grouping of hospitals for administrative and economic convenience resulted in:

> the separation of the matrons from policy making . . . but that this was not their only loss of power and status: they had also lost part of their empire. The grouping of hospitals had bureaucratised the administrative structure and had brought about further divisions of labour. Lay administrators and specialists were increasingly assuming responsibility for the linen rooms, laundries, female domestics, catering and other departments. The matrons found themselves left with responsibility only for the nurses and training schools.
>
> (White 1986b: 59)

White interprets the introduction of functional administration for 'non-nursing' services not as an overdue reform and a step towards modernizing nursing management but as contributing further to the matrons' erosion of power (White 1986b). White's argument however rests on two questionable assumptions. First, that the conditions which matrons enjoyed before the NHS were considerably more favourable than those that prevailed under the Health Service. Too little is known of the extent to which matrons participated in hospital administration before the NHS was established for comparisons to be drawn. Second, that the erosion of the matronly power had a negative impact upon the representation of 'nursing' interests on HMCs. This raises the contentious question of whose interests matrons did represent? The reservation of a block of seats exclusively for matrons on the GNC had earlier divided expert opinion on the Select Committee on the GNC in 1926 (House of Commons 1926). The Committee were unconvinced that matrons should be given privileged treatment to ensure their expertise was adequately represented and found in favour of free elections (House of Commons 1926). The Wood Committee some twenty-one years later in its examination of the nurse recruitment and training needs of the new NHS, identified the authoritarian attitudes of senior hospital nurses as a major cause of student nurse wastage (MoH *et al*. 1947). The assumption implicit in White's argument that matrons and rank and file interests were synonymous is questionable.

Costing concern

The one area where the importance of nursing could not be overlooked, however was in the NHS budget. Once it came into operation the financial implications of the new service horrified Labour and Conservative governments alike. Expenditure consistently outstripped estimates during the early years of the NHS. The process was led by the hospital sector and a large share of this was contributed to by nursing salaries. The early years of the health service saw an expansion in nursing establishments and a levelling up of salaries as a more uniform national approach to staffing and pay through Whitley Council was introduced, and an attempt was made to remedy the pre-war depression in this sector. As it became clear that inflation was not falling generally, however, Treasury orthodoxy dictated a close review of large public expenditure commitments. Within the NHS this meant the hospital sector and, within that, the large element represented by wages and salaries. These pressures became particularly acute with the outbreak of the Korean War and the need to finance Britain's United Nations effort (Webster 1985). Real wage increases for nurses, outstripping both the Retail and Prices Index and the Ministry of Labour's Index of Wages embarrassed a government which was seeking wage restraint in the private sector and was considering a freeze in the public sector (Webster 1985).

In the short term there was a debate about whether pay settlements should be included within the attempts to set ceilings on NHS expenditure, so that they would have to be met by other savings, or whether there should be automatic supplementation (Webster 1985). Aneurin Bevan, the Minister of Health, was also aware of the limited extent to which the Whitley machinery could be interfered with. But as the scale of their contribution to the costs of the NHS became apparent, nursing salaries presented an obvious target for containment. The result was a substantial long-term decline in the pay of nurses relative to that of other occupations (Smail and Gray 1982; Gray 1989). Although their wages were no longer depressed by the precarious solvency of the voluntary hospitals, nurses found themselves equally vulnerable to the chronic problems of maintaining public services in a stagnant national economy. Failing to achieve substantial economies by introducing prescription charges, the Ministry were forced to extract greater efficiency from existing resources by improved management against a background of periodic industrial unrest.

Management: mirage or miracle?

Management arrangements for hospitals remained an enduring concern for the MoH who referred the question of the internal administration of the hospital service to the CHSC for investigation in 1951. A report entitled the Internal Administration of the Hospital Service (Bradbeer Report) was produced in 1954 (MoH, CHSC 1954). The Bradbeer Committee added little that was new to the debate. Rights of direct participation were not recommended and nursing advisory bodies, at group level, were to have a majority nurse representation. The Bradbeer recommendations were permissive and seemed to have a minimal effect upon the participation of nurses in policy-making even at the periphery which may have reflected the difficulties of the centre in controlling the relatively autonomous Boards or alternatively the Boards imposing their views on HMCs.

Under the twin pressures of industrial mobilization and cost containment in the mid 1960s policy-makers turned to industrial and commercial models of controlling labour costs. Nursing as one of the largest groups of workers was inevitably singled out for special attention (Carpenter 1977). The Committee on Senior Nurse Staffing was the result (MoH *et al*. 1966). It was also the logical corollary of the Ministry's ambitious plans for hospital building to make good the deficiencies identified by the Guillebaud Committee established to investigate expenditure in the NHS (MoH 1956). The recommended structure in the Salmon Report was intended both to modernize nursing management to fit the new environments of the district general hospitals and to achieve a more efficient use of labour. Three tiers of administration were proposed:

1 Top management was to participate in the determination of hospital policy.
2 Middle management was responsible for translating plans into operational programmes for a particular sector, using clinical as well as managerial expertise.
3 First-line managers were to undertake executive functions thus ensuring that work was carried out according to plan.

A parallel scheme was later recommended by the Mayston Committee for local authority nursing services (DHSS *et al*. 1969).

For the first time nurses had a management system that could give them parity with other interests in the NHS. It was well adapted for the structure of the reorganized health service and anticipated much of the spirit of consensus management associated with the later 1974 reorganization.

Conclusions

What conclusions can be drawn from this review of policy participation by nurses in the early NHS? Firstly, it seems to have been assumed by the early NHS planners that nursing policy questions would be considered alongside those relating to health in general and that nurses would accommodate them-selves to whatever arrangements were made. There was no logical or consistent pattern to the participation of nurses in the health policy process whether at the centre or at the periphery. What is striking is the lack of effective action by the nursing organizations to lobby on behalf of their constituency. This not only contrasts markedly with organizations representing the medical profession but also with more assertive contemporary attitudes in nursing (Owen and Glennister 1990; Strong and Robinson 1990). The government was reluctant to magnify its problems by volunteering consultation to other groups but if nurses felt cheated or depressed by their position in the new arrangements, they were slow to register their protest to the arrangements.

The introduction of the NHS did not automatically enhance opportunities for nurses to participate in decision-making beyond the level accorded to groups of comparable status. Nurses were not the only group to feel disappointed by the arrangements offered to them. Labour and trade union interests themselves were not afforded the profile hoped for in the new administration (Webster 1988). Wider political concerns took precedence.

The NHS was established as a compromise between various vested interests from which a consensus emerged and which assumed a greater permanence than was originally envisaged (Webster 1988). The fragile nature of the consen-sus arguably inhibited the articulation of discontent by aggrieved groups and consequently sustained an artificially high level of support for the *status quo*. Fear of undermining the integrity and stability of the service arguably served to avert conflict and the need to absorb threatening elements into the of policy-making leadership. A different strategy was adopted in relation to the medical profession whose opposition to the service had to be purchased by co-option, arguably at the expense of other less powerful groups. Concessions to traditional interests meant that representational arrangements were worked out not on a rational basis but on the basis of political expediency and appeasement.

There was no inevitable reason for all nursing organizations to be pessimistic. Some did well out of representation particularly the RCN which had majority standing on the staff side of the newly established Whitley Councils. The pattern of representation on the Whitley Council reproduced arrangements on the Rushcliffe Committee and perpetuated tensions and rivalries between the RCN and unions (Gray 1989). The arrangement possibly reflected a preference on the part of the government for the RCNs' more hierarchical approach to pay policy rewarding higher grades and maintaining significant differentials between grades. It also promoted divisions that arguably sustained disunity within the occupation and illustrates the danger of referring to nursing 'inter-ests' as if these relate to a homogeneous community.

Representation may operate on a proportional or symbolic basis in which those elected or appointed hopefully reflect in miniature the cross-sectional views of their constituency. In the symbolic sense no attempt is made to take account of the size or range of interests potentially vested in one person. In either case representatives may act in accordance with or independently of a mandate. Like 'crisis' and 'policy', the term representation requires contextual definition.

The heterogeneity of nursing as an occupation means that different organizational objectives may be pursued by the various segments or specialisms which comprise the occupational community (Bucher and Strauss 1961). 'Segments' may be further stratified according to different levels of prestige and remuneration (Abbott 1988). 'Representation' needs to be critically considered in terms of representation of whom, for and by whom?

What conclusions might we draw about the relationship between 'crisis' and 'policy' in nursing? What role did nurses play in the 'crisis' of the early health service and to what extent was this seized upon as an opportunity to advance nursing interests? The shortage of nursing labour in the early years of the NHS never seriously undermined the future of the service, and the introduction of the NHS cannot be considered a 'crisis' in the sense that the identity of a social institution was threatened with disintegration, resulting in some massive rupture with tradition (Habermas 1976). The crisis of expenditure into which the service was plunged shortly after its inception was exacerbated by overdue increases in nurses' salaries but did not generate demands from nurses to enhance their policy-making profile or status.

The first significant attempt by a nursing organization to assert its own definition of nursing skill and division of labour was through the RCNs' sponsorship of the Platt Committee (RCN 1964; Dingwall *et al.* 1988). The reforms proposed by the Committee were linked to the perceived need to equip the nurse to assume the responsibilities of leadership. Leadership was never defined and the report failed to take account of trends in mainstream education and was further overtaken by the progress being made towards health service reorganization. The report was soon to become an anachronism. Even the subsequent establishment of the Briggs Committee in 1970 presupposed that, as in 1919 and 1946, both periods of alleged shortage of nursing labour, nursing would be reconstructed to fit the new system rather than being planned with it. Where changes deriving from an agenda set by nurses appears to have been successful this can usually be traced to a synchronization with wider organizational, and governmental concerns. The dissemination of two recent innovations, Project 2000 and primary nursing can be understood in this way (Dingwall *et al.* 1988).

Any assessment of the participation of nurses in policy-making involves a value-judgement as to what is acceptable representation under different conditions. No attempts have yet been made to identify the parameters by which 'success' or 'failure' could be 'measured'. Fundamental questions such as who represents which strand of nursing interests, what are the objectives of representatives and on what basis are strategies determined and operationalized are questions in need of research. Nurse leaders have been reluctant to define the nature of the 'expertise' they bring to policy decision-making to justify representation. The 'rationalist' culture of new model management means professional definitions of merit are no guarantee of participation for professionals in health care decision-making. The current 'crisis' in nursing, if one exists, can arguably be perceived as a 'crisis of confidence' in the capacity of nurses to legitimize their authority by their own efforts (Owen and Glennister 1990). If nurses feel beleaguered and their value system under threat, perhaps they need to seek more creative ways of expressing those values through innovative approaches to managing and delivering patient care.

7

Labour substitution and productivity in the care of the elderly

John Stilwell

The cost-effective deployment of appropriately qualified nursing staff is often claimed as the objective of nurse workforce planning. John Stilwell's chapter shows that the immense methodological problems involved in measuring outputs when trying to evaluate labour cost-effectiveness in a systematic and rigorous way can to some extent be side-stepped by focusing on process and the extent to which process goals are met. Using activity analysis in three homes and one ward caring for psychogeriatric patients, he finds that, as staff to client ratios increase, so a comparatively small proportion of the additional nursing time is devoted to 'positive' and direct activity with clients. In contrast, staff assigned to this task do devote a high proportion of time to it, leading John Stilwell to conclude that task assignment seems to compare favourably with the personalized care model of nursing when judged against certain desirable process objectives.

Introduction

The economic model most likely to be used to analyse the nursing process (in the non-technical sense), and to provide instruments of appraisal, could be baldly stated as: inputs → black-box → outputs. This simple conceptualization can be enormously powerful, because of its insistence on separate definitions of input and output. But its weakness is equally clear; the 'black box', in this case the nursing process, is, in a sense, left unmeasured; the only economically interesting characteristics are the value of the inputs, and the value of the output. Provided that patients get better faster, the process activities can be ignored.

The long-term care of elderly patients with deterioration of mental function is one of the most difficult areas of nursing to appraise within a conceptual framework which deals with outputs of the nursing process, as well as inputs. First the medical cause–effect relationships may be imperfectly understood. Second, the links between *process* and outcome may not be obvious. Clean sheets and a well-made bed may seem very important to some patients, but not to others. In principle, the value of these activities can be partly assessed by asking patients, but such assessment is easier if the process has some (perhaps slight) link to outcome: for example, clean sheets and a well-made bed may reduce the probability of cross-infection or bed-sores. Third, activities relating to the psychological well-being of the patient are important activities but are more difficult areas in which to develop process proxies for outcome because, quite simply, appropriate psychological support is more difficult to determine than appropriate physical support. A dirty dressing should always be changed; but to some patients quietness and withdrawal may be their own coping mechanism. So process measures are more difficult to employ with confidence – but although they are more difficult, they are nevertheless in principle possible.

These difficulties have led to the development of a list of objectives for care which is closely linked to the standard methods of assessing psychogeriatric dependency. These methods are usually simple and fairly arbitrary algorithms, summing weighted staff perceptions of patients and patients' scores on various tests of memory and intelligence. Few units, however, use such instruments systematically to monitor the quality of care, probably because they are not sufficiently refined to capture the very small positive changes which are all that can be hoped for after the quite substantial dependency fluctuations that take place at the start of a patient's stay in a nursing home or ward (Sixsmith *et al.* 1990).

There are also many cases where an improvement upon one dimension has to be set against a deterioration upon another; or where (and this is the commonest) the assessment is too difficult to make.

Yet, despite this apparent insuperable obstacle, there is a clear way through to economic appraisal. It may not be possible to measure objective outcome, but it is certainly possible to measure the degree to which the professional carers meet their own process goals. Thus the external evaluator can confine his or her measurement of output to simple indicators such as mortality, and concentrate upon examining whether the professional stated aims of the care decision makers are actually being achieved.

The professional model of care

The predominant professional model of primary nursing care is well summarized by Brocklehurst and Andrews (1987):

> Current nursing practice is now based on the nursing process. This involves personalized nursing in that individual nurses are responsible for the total nursing care of small groups of patients – with whose problems and personalities they may become completely familiar. . . . We believe this is absolutely right for geriatric patients at all stages of care (acute, rehabilitation and long stay).

The homes

Against this background, the DoH asked the University Department of Psychiatry at Liverpool, and the Health Services Research Centre at Warwick, to study three new homes for the elderly mentally ill which were set up in 1984 under the Special Medical Development Programme.

These homes were set up in order to provide care with three different types of staffing arrangement. They were all generously staffed, but with more untrained than in the NHS, so the two crucial differences between them and other, conventional wards were the level of staffing and the ratio of qualified to unqualified staff.

Alpha is operated by social services, with care staff employed by the local authority, but with a team of supporting workers from a number of disciplines, most of whom are employed by the health authority. Beta is operated by the health authority, and run more or less as if it were a small separate hospital, except that the nurse in charge is not fully independent and must refer some decisions to a senior nurse in the hospital a quarter of a mile away. Gamma is also run by a health authority, but the nurse in charge operates much as a social services officer in charge. However, at Gamma most of the staff are unqualified general assistants, combining a caring and domestic role. Day care takes place only at Gamma.

All experimental sites operated a primary nurse or key worker system. However, these systems were radically different from what is conventionally understood as primary nursing in that the care plans for residents were made by the members of the teams jointly, and in some cases, in the absence of the qualified

Table 7.1 Staffing data

Home	Clients	Qualified staff (wte)	Unqualified staff (wte)	Qualified to unqualified staff	Qualified staff to clients	Unqualified staff to clients	Total staff to clients
Alpha	21	9	18	0.5	0.43	0.86	1.29
Beta	22	11.25	14	0.8	0.51	0.64	1.15
Gamma	20 res	7	18	0.4	0.35	0.9	1.25
	13 day	3	5.25	0.6	0.23	0.4	0.63
CC Ward	23	9	8.5	1.1	0.39	0.37	0.76

staff or even – as a deliberate policy – by the unqualified staff. Nor were these staff, although technically unqualified, very experienced; they were young, inexperienced but highly motivated.

In order to provide a comparison from outside the experimental setting, we also looked at a modern but conventional hospital continuing care psychogeriatric ward.

Staffing data on the homes is shown in Table 7.1 which indicates that Alpha had the highest staff/client ratio and that the continuing care ward (the comparison unit) was the worst off, not only in staff per client but also in observed records per staff. This is because absenteeism was higher during the study period than in the other units.

The qualified/unqualified ratios were very different between the three experimental units and the comparison unit, being much higher in the last (although average for a NHS long-stay geriatric ward). In fact, Gamma has subsequently – partly in response to the regrading exercise for nursing staff – reduced even further the number of qualified staff.

Gamma is different from the other units in that it has adopted completely the generic worker model. Its staff carry out almost all the domestic work as well as caring for the residents. This distorts the comparison with the other units, where the domestic work is under the control of the domestic supervisor, and carried out on site. Beta employed about 10.5 wte domestic, catering, estates and portering staff. Alpha employed 4 wte. We have no such breakdown for the comparison unit. Beta is on three floors (two for the residents) and is larger than Alpha, but the enormous difference between 4 and 10.5 staff remains unexplained. However, the first question raised is whether it is consistent with the professional, primary, model for care staff to perform domestic duties, and the second is whether it is cost effective. We return to these questions later.

Table 7.2 shows data on patient dependency in the homes. Dependency, whether measured by Cape (Pattie and Gilleard 1979) or the Crichton Royal (Wilkin and Jolley 1979) was highest in the ward, second highest in Beta, then Gamma, and lowest at Alpha. However, this difference did not appear so

Table 7.2 Client dependency data (results are expressed as percentages of clients)

Home	Cape (survey)					Immobile	Crichton Royal		
	A	B	C	D	E	%	High Dep.	Med Dep.	Low Dep.
Alpha ·	6	6	32	50	6	0	0	55	45
Beta	–	–	–	–	–	27	32	63	5
Gamma	–	–	–	–	–	5	5	69	21
CC Ward	0	5	5	10	80	23	45	40	15

marked to research staff who knew each home, and dependencies at Alpha may have been relatively under-reported because of the ethos among the staff at Alpha who were perhaps prone to minimize the behaviour problems of residents.

Both Beta and the ward had about a quarter of residents who were totally immobile. Each of these facilities had originally gained some of their residents from a decanting exercise from a large mental illness hospital, and this accounted for the highly dependent states of some clients.

The study

We undertook an activity analysis study for a complete week in each home and the comparison unit, in order to find out what tasks were performed, by whom, and with which clients. This information could then be interpreted in the light of each home's objectives, and it could also be used to see how evenly, or unevenly, the care was distributed between staff and among all the clients, and whether any particular type of client laid an especially heavy burden upon staff. It could also be combined with information from observational studies, and to a certain extent ethnographic work, in order to triangulate upon certain key areas of importance to health facility planners.

Two available methods for collecting systematic data on staff activities were observation by the survey team, and self-reporting. Observation is more objective, but suffers from the theoretical drawback that the observers might not thoroughly understand, and might accordingly misinterpret, the activities performed. For example, without knowing the detailed care plan for a particular client, it might not be obvious to the observer whether an interaction such as help with feeding was routine or specially planned for that client. This disadvantage should not be exaggerated – the classification of most activities is fairly clear.

Self-reporting is less objective, but more sensitive.

The most important difference, however, is the relative information productivity of the two systems; self-reporting yields about 4–6 times as much information per member of research staff involved.

We therefore decided to undertake the main study by means of self-reporting, and to perform some smaller observational studies in order to test for consistency. The main study is used as material for this chapter; the observational studies were consistent with the main study.

Following a one-week pilot study, at Alpha, a diary form was designed which was used in the main study.

The main 'ingredient' which we wished to capture was whatever characteristic of an observation could be used to distinguish those events that the care staff decision makers would classify as furthering the care objectives of the home. This was in accordance with our principle of evaluating performance according to the degree with which the homes' own objectives were met.

All the homes had developed quite detailed written aims and objectives. After discussion within the homes, we decided that the special aim of the homes – over and above such aims as good routine health and comfort care the provision of which might be seen, in our terms, as a constraint to satisfy rather than an objective to maximize – was to deliver that type of care that is the most difficult for even the most loving of relatives to deliver consistently in the home setting. This is to stimulate the minds and engage the interests of the clients.

We termed this type of care 'Positive' care. It is close in concept to 'Engagement' (Blunden and Kushlick 1974), although it carries with it the additional implication that the subject is interacting with a member of care staff, whereas it is possible to be 'engaged' on one's own, or solely with another resident.

The other two permissible characterizations of staff–resident interactions were 'Demanding' and 'Routine'. An event was Demanding if a resident 'sidetracked' the member of staff in such a way that the staff member's planned activities were disrupted in a non-trivial way. Everything else was defined as Routine.

Each member of care staff, including members of supporting disciplines such as occupational therapy or social work, was given a diary in which the week was divided into quarter-hour slots. She was asked to describe each quarter-hour period in the following terms:

1 Was it with or not with clients?
2 If with, with whom, and was it Positive, Demanding or Routine?
3 If not with, was it a Task, Administration or a Break?
4 If at night, was it Observation?

And a brief description of the activity.

Table 7.3 Summary of observations

Home	No. of observations	Observations	
		With clients (%)	Not with clients (%)
Alpha	3795	2010 (53)	1785 (47)
Beta	3337	2123 (64)	1214 (36)
Gamma			
Day	941	533 (57)	408 (43)
Residential	3009	1687 (56)	1322 (44)
Ward	2288	1399 (61)	889 (39)

The results

Table 7.3 shows the total number of observations for the three units, and the percentage split between time spent 'with' or 'not with' clients.

Table 7.4 shows the percentage of time each staff group spent 'with clients', indicating that Alpha's trained staff spend the lowest proportion of time with residents. Beta has the highest proportions of staff with clients for all except night staff.

Table 7.4 also reveals a very large difference between the ratios for Other staff at Alpha and Beta. This category comprises different types of staff at the two homes. At Alpha it comprises the multi-disciplinary team, including Occupational Therapist, Doctor, Community Psychiatric Nurse and other specialists on a sessional basis. At Beta it covers only Activity Organizers, who are untrained staff performing a diversional therapy role.

We divided not-with-clients records into four categories, Administration, Task, Break and Observation at night. The main category of staff activity not undertaken with clients is the classification 'Task'. Tasks can be subdivided into housekeeping and professional/clerical, such as report writing. Within these subdivisions we formed further categories; within professional/clerical we have supervision, handover, report writing, other writing, discussions and meetings. Within housekeeping we have tidying, washing/laundry, cleaning,

Table 7.4 Percentage of time spent with clients, by staff group

Home	Trained	Untrained	Night	Other
Alpha	38	71	–	40
Beta	62	71	55	85
Gamma	49	59	56	–
Ward	59	63	61	–

Table 7.5 Breakdown of time spent not with clients

	Alpha	*Beta*	*Gamma*	*Ward*
Total not-with-clients	1785	1214	1730	889
Administration	195	128	208	112
Tasks				
(a) Professional/clerical				
Supervision	67	14	0	3
Handover	252	140	130	224
Report writing	214	188	25	3
Other writing	56	19	33	3
Discussion	192	36	7	66
Meeting	105	19	70	17
Sub-total	1081 (61)	544 (45)	473 (27)	428 (48)
(b) Housekeeping				
Tidying	53	9	11	23
Washing/laundry	74	14	237	28
Cleaning	17	8	90	12
Ironing	0	0	26	0
General domestic	2	0	68	0
Sub-total	146 (8)	31 (3)	432 (25)	63 (7)
(c) Residual	320 (18)	220 (18)	404 (23)	269 (30)
Break	238 (13)	274 (23)	363 (21)	109 (12)
Observation	0 (0)	145 (12)	58 (3)	20 (2)

ironing, and general domestic. There is also a residual category for such items as 'collecting prescription and buying a necklace for resident'. The breakdown of records into these categories is given in Table 7.5. We have subtotalled Administration with Professional/clerical because of their similarity. Column percentages are given in brackets.

It is immediately apparent that Alpha stands on its own, with a heavy professional/clerical load, equivalent to about eight full person days. Gamma has far more housekeeping than the others. This is because the staff at Gamma also perform the jobs done in the other homes by domestic staff. Other noteworthy points are the low domestic loads at Beta and the Ward, and the low overall figure at the Ward.

Returning to time spent with clients, we wished to look in more detail at the division of time between 'Positive', 'Demanding', and 'Routine' care, as defined earlier. In particular we wished to investigate two questions; first, did Positive care increase with staff numbers, secondly, as total staff increased, did Positive care increase at an increasing rate – that is, as more staff came on duty, was any increase greater than the average proportion of Positive care? To

Table 7.6 Breakdown of time spent with clients

	Alpha	*Beta*	*Gamma*	*Ward*
Total with clients	2010	2123	2220	1399
Positive	288	240	501	202
Demanding	252	255	201	193
Routine	1470	1628	1518	1004
Total staff to client ratio	1.29	1.15	1.25	0.76

look at this question we considered both comparisons between units, and within each unit since there were different staffing levels at different times.

The 'between units' analysis was simple. Alpha had most staff and second highest number of Positives, Gamma had the next highest number of staff, and most Positives, Beta had the third highest number of staff and the third highest number of Positives, and the ward had least of each. These results are shown in Table 7.6 and Figure 7.1.

To see whether an increase in the number of staff on duty within each unit would lead to an increase in the amount of Positive care, it was necessary to make two adjustments to the data sets. First, we needed to test and, if needed, correct for serial correlation. (This means that we could not proceed as if every quarter-hour observation was unaffected by the previous observation; for

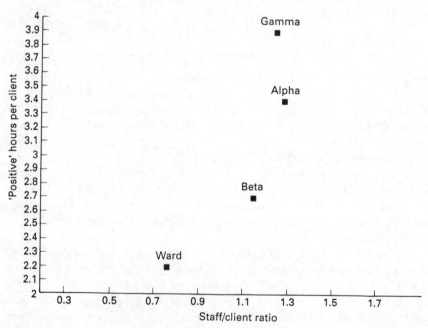

Figure 7.1 Relation between staffing levels and amount of positive care

example, if three Occupational Therapists came on duty for two hours with the aim of concentrating on Positive care, the Positive count would be high for all eight observations. However, this would not give us eight times the information received in the first observation.)

Secondly, we needed to remove observations which would tend to mislead. During mealtimes staffing is usually high, but without much intention or possibility of giving a great deal of Positive care. We accordingly excluded mealtimes from the within-unit analysis. At night, staffing is low and Positive care also low. Including night-time observations would have added spurious strength to any correlation observed between the numbers of staff on duty and the number of Positive episodes.

We performed simple linear regressions of the number of staff undertaking Positive care upon the total number of staff present, correcting for serial correlation by the Durbin Watson method (Neter and Wasserman 1974). Serial correlation was high and positive in all four sites. The coefficient of determination after correction was about two-thirds of its value before correction.

After correction it was 0.45 at Gamma, 0.41 at Alpha, 0.1 at Beta and 0.1 at the Ward. The slope coefficients were 0.24 at Gamma, 0.25 at Alpha and 0.14 at Beta (all these were significant at the 0.025 level; Gamma and Alpha at the 0.001 level). At the Ward, the slope was 0.1, but not significant at the 0.05 level.

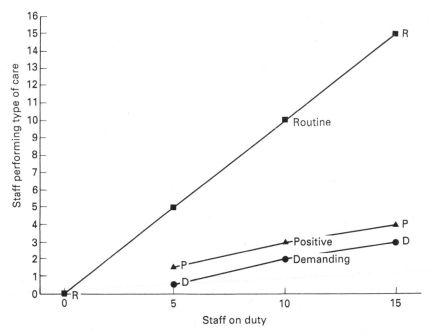

Figure 7.2 Proportion of three types of care as numbers of staff on duty increase

All the equations showed positive intercepts with the axis along which staff numbers were measured. This implies that at very low levels of staff no appreciable amount of Positive care was undertaken – this is consistent with common sense. It also means that the proportion of care given as Positive increases as staff numbers increase.

The slope coefficient of about a quarter at Alpha and Gamma means that as extra staff come on, about a quarter of their time is spent on Positive care, or, more accurately, that either this is the case, or the extra staff release staff already present to perform more Positive care. Overall (again, excluding night and meal times), 16 per cent of total staff time is spent on Positive care.

The relationship between increasing numbers of staff on duty and the type of care performed is summarized in Figure 7.2.

Conclusions

What, then are the main conclusions to draw from these figures?

First, we see that the majority of direct patient care – that is, time with clients – is performed by untrained staff. If we compare the best staffed of the experimental homes – Alpha – with the Ward, we see that they each possessed the same number of qualified staff. Yet 62 per cent of time of qualified staff at Alpha was spent on administrative and other non-direct-care duties, compared with 41 per cent at the Ward. There was, therefore, a substitution of untrained for trained staff. This was true for Gamma also, but not Beta.

We have already explained that Gamma employed no domestic staff, but that all hotel functions were performed by the generic care workers, employed on nursing auxiliary grades. The activity study gave us data to assess the simple economics of this, although the policy was not in place to save money, but as part of a total philosophy of care. We found that the hotel work undertaken was the equivalent of three and a half full-time staff. This was less than Alpha, and much less than Beta; given that Gamma had the highest workload, this policy was probably cost effective, even allowing for the fact that nursing auxiliaries are paid more than domestic staff. But we have to comment that this policy, justified in non-economic terms partly as an efficient method of stress-buffering, and partly in terms of holistic care, was not particularly popular among the staff who tended to complain that it was a waste of their acquired skills.

To turn now to the real essence of the study: what was the productivity of the extra labour at the three experimental homes? Look again at Figure 7.2. There were an average of 9 staff on daytime duty at Alpha, compared with 4.8 at the Ward. But of these additional 4.2 staff at Alpha 3.2 were engaged in extra Routine care and only 1 in extra Positive care. Yet we have no reason to believe that the standard of Routine care at the Ward was in any way unsatisfactory. No short cuts to hygiene care were adopted; all residents received appropriate nutritional care; there was a constant supply of tea, coffee and biscuits. Physical needs were monitored and attended to. So even if we assume a very considerable sampling error, we are still left with the conclusion that we could have expected far more extra, specialist, Positive care than was actually delivered. Daytime resources were almost doubled, but this resulted in only a 25 per cent increase in Positive care.

So the crucial question is, is the failure of an increase in staffing levels to deliver relatively more Positive care due to the lack of training of the staff, or the way in which care was organized, or the very nature of the job?

The conclusion most palatable to the proponents of the professional paradigm of nursing (Robinson *et al.* 1989) would be that this is exactly what would have been expected from so unbalanced an expansion in resources. But we do not feel that this explanation is correct. Primary nursing, which is part of the professional model, was in place at all units; the qualified staff were perfectly aware of up-to-date thinking in their professions. Yet the qualified staff, apart from the nurses or officers in charge, were just as likely to take part in manual, not-with-clients activities (termed 'associated' care in some systems) as the unqualified staff. Thus, there was no obvious evidence that a professional training would make a member of staff more likely to deliver additional 'Positive' care.

Moreover, although most staff spent less than a quarter of their time on Positive care, there were two categories of staff who spent about three-quarters of their time on Positive care. These were the staff at Beta and Gamma who were employed as activity organizers, or Occupational Therapy Aides (OTA). There was a corresponding member of staff at the Ward, who was the OTA in the Day Hospital which two residents attended occasionally. (These records were included in the study.)

These staff, five in number, and only part-time, were unqualified but highly motivated and many activities revolved around them although they accounted for only a small part of the Homes' budget. Their job descriptions concentrated on the specific Positive activities of Reality Orientation, Occupational and Diversional Therapy, and excluded help with physical caring activities.

All the homes subscribed to the philosophy that the care of persons with dementia-like illnesses is a skill which can be taught in the manner of an apprenticeship, with emphasis on practical aspects, but without ignoring the necessary intellectual – and, indeed especially, the moral – content. Yet this sat uneasily with an equal acknowledgement of the professionalizing nature of nursing and residential social work. The observed facts of the situation are that, to return to Brocklehurst's phraseology, when 'individual nurses (were) responsible for the total nursing care of small groups of patients' – and where these patients suffer from that most stressful condition, dementia, a care model that includes a considerable element of task assignment appeared more likely to maximize Positive care than a model that relies on personalized care alone.

8

Care, work and carework: A synthesis?

Nicky James

The issues that Nicky James writes about in this chapter resonate in policy terms at several levels. First, by contrasting domestic care and health care, links are made between ideology and policy, and issues of the gender division of caring work and of occupation are raised. Second, a hospice study is used to illustrate the gap between the aspirations inherent in policy-making and the day-to-day work which adjusts these ideals. This implies a series of transformations through which ideologies of care become modified by policy-making and further qualified during practical implementation. Care policy is thereby explained as merely one aspect of a broader social process. Finally, Nicky James illustrates the need for conceptual clarity when analysing the problem of defining nursing care. In identifying the complex interaction between the invisible outcomes of good care and the visible outcomes of physical tasks and routines, and highlighting the gaps between the ideals and the reality of care, Nicky James contributes to a critique of nursing's opportunities and constraints in health care provision.

Introduction

Nursing is in danger of appearing to claim a monopoly on caring. Our use of 'care' implies that we have forgotten the millions of skilled, unpaid carers, as well as the waged carers in the voluntary sector, social workers, home helps, child minders and probation officers. Interestingly, social policy research is similarly myopic, ignoring analyses of nursing care (Graham 1991) with the result that nursing policy and social policy fail to learn from each other. So although 'care' is highly symbolically significant and vitally affects policy issues, understanding of the process of 'caring' is partial and narrowly focused. In recent years nurses' occupational identity has increasingly and pervasively been explained as that of carers (Leininger 1984). Caring has become a foundation philosophy of nursing in diploma and degree courses so that future generations of nurses will perceive 'care' as being fundamental to their craft and the services they offer.

Clearly 'caring' has resonated at a personal and professional level with the aspirations of many of us involved in nursing, giving impetus to its inclusion in our images of ourselves and becoming embodied in the service standards we are increasingly setting. Yet Armstrong (1983b) claimed that 'care' in the sense of dynamic relationships has only recently been introduced into nursing – superimposed on a history of hygiene and order (Davies 1976, 1977).

If we intend to make 'caring' central to our professional identities, to make it part of our contribution to health outcomes, then we need to examine our motives for doing so and the intended and unintended consequences of our claims. Questions of motivation and consequence require an historical and contemporary context. Undoubtedly gender, occupational status and other forms of stratification will be central to the analysis.

We also need to consider the constraints within which we develop this newly formalized element of nursing, the knowledge, attitude and skills, so that we are conscious of the limitations of our work. I believe that without examining these processes we will not be able to generate a wise critique of nursing care within health services. As a result we may be disappointed when nurses' overclaims leave us vulnerable to failure in the policies and practices we develop.

My contribution to this major debate is an examination of the gap between the rhetoric and the practice of 'care' as perceived by nurses at a hospice and analysed in terms of 'care', 'work' and 'carework'. The chapter will be divided into two main sections. Firstly I shall explore two ideologies of care – domestic care and nursing care. Secondly I will use the hospice study to explain the terms 'care', 'work' and 'carework' in a dual sense as both nursing practice and analytic categories. In conclusion I question whether there is, or should be a synthesis between 'care' and 'work' to become 'carework'.

Care as ideology

'Care' and 'caring' are phrases that are currently so over-used as to be meaning-less. Politicians use them to give a personal flavour to policies designed as blanket measures to deal with national troubles; commercial and industrial employers use them to convey their concern for individual employees; and 'lacking in care' is used as a tabloid criticism of public services such as children's homes and even prisons.

Despite the pervasiveness of 'care' in our lives, academic analysis of 'the family', 'work' and 'organization' have failed until very recently to consider the social relations through which ideologies of care are produced and reproduced. As Graham (1983) showed, until feminist writers began to look at women's contribution to social production and reproduction, divisions between academic subjects, and between academics and practitioners, obscured rather than illuminated our understanding of care. Ironically, terms introduced by feminists, and co-opted to analyse 'care', add to already existing conceptual difficulties. 'Private' and 'public' are used by feminists to distinguish the domestic domain from the world of paid employment, while in policy terms 'private' provision of care refers not to unpaid care at home, but to its antithesis – paid care for profit. Similarly, the term 'informal care', used to distinguish domestic care from public provision, seems to imply a casual, secondary form of care subject to chance agreements, rather than the numerically, socially and materially dominant form of care upon which current community policies depend and build.

But regardless of commercialism, academics, and the current fashion of 'caring', it is still in families, at home, that as a society we invest our greatest faith in the importance and centrality of care. *Caring for People* (DoH *et al.* 1989a) sought to redress the balance of caring provision away from institutions and back into 'community'. Though there are criticisms of the outcomes, the policy undoubtedly builds on a traditional assumption of family-type care being best (Dalley 1988). Even as adults it is still a truism that we all need to be cared for and 'family' may still be first port of call whether we need someone to listen to our woes and successes, or to give advice when the car breaks down. In this sense then we are all both carers and cared for. Thus the category of 'carer' is one that is relative to time and circumstance, and not merely to paid occupation.

The breadth of family contributions to care means that 'family' is used by society in general and health carers in particular as an ideal-type, a form of 'pure' care. Even if 'family' is adapted for professional and service circumstances, its significance in understanding the gender division of labour offers important insights into the ways gender affects employment and employees – which, of course, includes nurses (for example see Pahl 1984; Sharpe 1984; Dex 1985; Hearn and Parkin 1987). Since gender relations also permeate the content and delivery of health services an understanding of the influence of an ideal of family care on nursing services is vital (Gamarnikow 1978; Leeson and Gray 1978; Salvage 1985; Webb 1985; Stacey 1988; James 1989). It is not that all nurses believe that it is appropriate to emulate family-type care, rather that, like it or not, it is an historical underpinning of the way health 'care' services are provided. For this reason, comparisons between family or domestic care and health care are illuminating, highlighting similarities and differences of structure and process.

A dictionary definition of ideology is as 'beliefs, attitudes and opinions which form sets, whether tightly or loosely related' (Abercrombie *et al.* 1984), and by comparing the sets of beliefs underpinning domestic and health care we can highlight similarities and differences of structure and process. As Dalley notes in relation to social care:

> . . . a particular view of the family and the expected roles of its various members underlies a whole range of policies – especially, but not exclusively, policies related to caring.
>
> (Dalley 1988: 20)

Domestic care

For the purposes of this essay, family care is used synonymously with domestic care. Social science definitions of family highlight it as an 'institution' concerned with social regulation (Mann 1983), but an historian gave a more lively definition when he described eighteenth-century families as being:

> the elemental unit of living and dying, reproduction and socialisation, education and business, love and hate.
>
> (Porter 1982: 160)

Though nowadays health staff standardly intervene in many of these processes, historically, care in western society has primarily been a family duty with the home the main locus of care. The change from rural to a predominantly industrial society, caused changes in patterns of family life. The separation of paid labour into the rigidly timetabled workplace accentuated an already strong gender division of labour, so that in the twentieth century in the west, for the most part, family care has meant women's care. Women in their capacity as 'homemakers' are held responsible not just for the care of their children, but for the care, in its broadest sense, of their family – the needs of their husbands and the nursing of dependent relatives. It was in 1956 that Parsons and Bales (quoted in Oakley 1974) restated women's roles as being 'nurturant' and 'expressive' in comparison with the instrumental 'work' roles of men.

Though we know that 55 per cent of women with dependent children work (*Central Statistical Office* 1991), and despite studies which include male carers (Bytheway 1987; Ungerson 1987; Arber and Gilbert 1989), both the ideology and the practice of women as carers remain strong (Ungerson 1983; Brook and Davis 1985).

The intimacy that is characteristic of family care arises as the result of sustained relationships. The objectivity or 'distance' required in professional health care staff would be a criticism if applied to the way women care for dependants at home.

As carers and cared for have known each other over time, often for many years, and in different circumstances, they know each other's strengths and weaknesses. The personal knowledge which is learned through shared lives means that domestic care relations develop within the context of physical and emotional familiarity with people and of place. Although much has been written in the USA and Britain about child abuse and granny battering, making it clear that family relations are far from unproblematic, this has not undermined the fundamental assumption that family care is best (*Feminist Review* 1988).

A further point to be made about domestic care is that the roles of 'cared for' and 'carer' are not necessarily readily identifiable. Increasing numbers of carers are themselves likely to be in receipt of some form of 'care'. As Kirschling (1986) observes 'the frail (are) caring for the frail' and in studies of the terminally ill it has been noted that one in four of the main domestic carers of hospice patients were over 75 (Wilkes 1986).

In general, then, domestic care takes place in familiar surroundings, with familiar people, where carer and cared for may reciprocate or exchange roles over time, and where, at least in rhetoric, it is often regarded as women's work. In organizational terms the family, though small, serves myriad functions of which health care is merely one.

Health care

The health sector is vague about its use of 'care', with the journal *Care Science and Practice*, published by The Society for Tissue Viability, consisting solely of biochemical research, while hospices have long used the phrase 'total care' to cover social, psychological, spiritual and physical care.

Current debates over appropriate care policies have a long precedent, as does public provision of care for the poor and sick with religious orders providing extensive hospice shelter for travellers and the sick poor across Europe in medieval times (Stoddard 1979). Rates were being levied to support the poor in Norwich in 1549 (Stacey 1988), and one in five families were in receipt of poor relief in the eighteenth century (Porter 1982). People also bought their own health care as over centuries an array of healers offered their services in return for money, goods and services (Stacey 1988; Porter 1989).

It has been argued that it was progress in the study of anatomy and philosophical changes in beliefs about pain during the Enlightenment, together with the effects of a capitalist labour market which laid the foundations of modern health care (Doyal 1979; Porter 1982). The result was that during the course of the nineteenth century practices changed substantially. Influenced by the developing biomedical approach to sickness, specialization and professionalization grew. The emphasis was on cure: women healers were usurped (Donnison 1977); there was a change from 'unskilled, untrustworthy nurses to a kind that were useful and efficient' (Williams 1980); and increasingly there was a form of selectivity through which some forms of sickness became subject to workplace, institutional care.

Although since the Second World War chronic disease has replaced acute illness the 'acute-care mentality' approach to illness continues to direct and shape health services (Strauss *et al.* 1985). Doctors' skills and knowledge are founded upon a scientific approach to medicine, based on biological divisions into specialization, and a central interest in body malfunction. The very nature of medical inquiry generates a sense of distance and objectivity, and nurses, the carers most directly associated with the patients, have also been taught until relatively recently that it is professional to remain distanced from 'the patient' (Hockey 1979; Armstrong 1983a, b).

The NHS, despite its name, has concentrated on illness rather than wellness, and though there is government commitment to redress the balance toward health prevention we have over 100 years of history of 'illness' services to overcome and to adjust through the retraining of personnel.

Health care, like family care, has been analysed in terms of its controlling function (Foucault 1976; Turner 1987), and historically nursing too takes on this role (Dean and Bolton in Davies 1980; essays in Hutter and Williams 1981; Dingwall *et al.* 1988). Post-war developments in health care extended clinical influence and territory to include the well in addition to the ill and with it the possibility of extending its controlling function (Armstrong 1983a; Arney and Bergen 1983). Within this context, which included the extension of 'team-work', nursing too had an opportunity to develop and extend its remit (Wouters 1990).

While nursing history is not synonymous with medical history, we would be foolish to ignore the directions in which nursing was led by medicine from the hospital based education after Elizabeth Fry's intervention in the 1830s, through to the struggles for registration in 1919 (Bellaby and Oribabor 1980; Williams 1980). Now there are debates as to whether nurses should extend their roles to take on diagnostic and technical work which has previously been doctors', or whether we work to develop and expand our own craft and skills, but in either case, nursing is intimately bound in its health care provision to its relations with doctors.

So what about the introduction of care into nursing? Literature shows that individuals' intentions to 'care' have been longstanding, even if the education and the system appeared to divert the aspiration (Brittain 1984; Wilson-Barnett 1988; Law Harrison 1990). Nursing histories have tended to focus on hospital nursing (Abel-Smith 1960; Maggs 1983), but even where the sweep has been broader (Davies 1980; Dingwall *et al.* 1988) 'care' still makes no appearance either as a main heading or sub-heading, in the indices. Is it then that the concept is too big, too nebulous, or, as Armstrong has implied, too recent a concern to be included? While there is debate on the specifics of Armstrong's assessment of the newness of 'care' in nursing, some of the current catch phrases such as 'holistic care', individual patient care, personalized care, 'total care' are, historically speaking, either making a come-back or of recent intro-duction (Wilson-Barnett 1988). Undoubtedly there are elements of 'care' which are being given greater attention so that, for example counselling skills are being taught to pre- and post-registration staff in ways unconsidered fifteen years ago, and books are available on nursing and spiritual care which were unheard of in the 1970s and much of the 1980s.

So nursing 'care' is changing within the broader context of post-war changes in health care which inevitably influence nurses' opportunities both to develop and implement ideas. I am also arguing that nursing has taken many cues from medicine – albeit unwillingly – and that, as in the family, gender relations have been a key aspect of job demarcation. The health care organization within which nurses work is a system of specialist paid labour subject to demarcation by craft (different types of nurse, doctor, manager and ancillary staff). The recipients of health care, patients, usually seek attention in specialized buildings – the workplace of the health care employees.

In broad terms, key contrasts between domestic and health care are that the former is privately arranged and fulfilled, often by unpaid women, in 'the home' which also serves other functions, while the latter is the result of special training, carried out in single-purpose, health services building by employees working in return for status, wages and power under hierarchical organizations.

Developing analyses of 'caring work'

In the summaries of domestic and health care, I have suggested that they have been derived from separate social histories with different meanings and expectations. Although practical, theoretical and evaluative means exist for understanding a whole series of 'work' relations and activities (Eldridge 1980; Holland 1980), it remains hard to account for a major aspect of service pro-vision, that is 'caring work'.

The difficulty of creating an analytic framework which can accommodate public and private (e.g. domestic) care, waged and unwaged workers, and emo-tional and physical labour, is reflected in the difficulties nurses are currently having in conveying the essence of nursing. Nurses have brought to the work-place the unpaid, domestic skills learned during what Oakley refers to as 'the long-apprenticeship' (Oakley 1974), and developed the craft of nursing from that foundation.

Accepting that there are new influences on the demand and opportunities for 'caring' work and its associated skills, it is interesting to consider ways in which the rhetoric has been implemented in changing practice, and where the rhetoric remains just that – an aspiration. It was with this question in mind that I first started studying hospices in the early 1980s. The concerns developed from my disbelief at what was being claimed for and by nurses, when it seemed that we were in danger of believing that our prescriptive ideals were synonymous with our practice, rather than being an adaptation of them. It seems likely that my concern then about the gaps between ideals and practice is still pertinent as we attempt to grapple with standard setting in the rapidly changing world of British health care (Flynn 1990; Strong and Robinson 1990; Sheaff 1991) for, as Ungerson has pointed out 'policy is personal' (Ungerson 1987).

The research

The hospice study from which the categories of care, work and carework were generated consisted of three periods of participating observation, one month in one hospice (as part of a course), two months on a hospital medical ward, and five months at a second hospice. During these periods I worked as a nurse on the shift system, and the observations were complemented by 'tape conversations' with the staff of the second hospice and visits to other hospice units (James 1986). The main research report focuses on the second hospice, which I refer to as Byresfold.

The research questions posed were:

1 Does the unit achieve the idealistic aims set for hospices – that is the delivery of 'total care' (social, psychological, physical and spiritual), with the family as the unit of care?
2 How do the nurses manage their care relative to their ideals?

Three striking observations on the nursing implementation of hospice principles arose directly from the fieldwork and taped conversations. First was the clarity with which the nurses explained the purpose of 'their unit' which tallied closely with the delivery of 'total care'. This point is currently relevant as wards and units develop their 'philosophies' and complementary 'standards'. Secondly, they noted the gap between their expectations of the care they felt they should give and the care they did give – the transposition of their principles into practice; and thirdly, despite noting the gap and giving good explanations for why it existed, there was little attempt during the research period to draw conclusions from it, or to change the aims or the practices.

It was the nurses' use of the categories 'care' and 'work' which I adopted and built on for the study. Though 'care' and 'work' are both necessary and complementary parts of a whole, the nurses associated each with different clusters of meanings and expectations. They used them as tools for analysing the gap between their ideals and their practice. 'Carework' was the term I developed both to describe a category of practice, and a means of analysis. So the nurses *explained* their care of the dying in terms of a tension between care and work, but, I suggest, they *practised* their care of the dying in terms of 'carework'.

Care

Observations

'Care' has been a fundamental part of hospice help from medieval times (Stoddard 1979) and fits the modern ethos of hospice services, that is to provide 'eu-thanatos' – the 'good death'. The unanimity with which the Byresfold nurses (who included enrolled nurses and auxiliaries) described the unit's purpose as being to 'give good care' was interesting, though most had not read any formal research on care or on hospices. The following quotation, which includes many aspects of 'total care', comes from a 19-year-old, temporary auxiliary nurse:

> Well the purpose of this unit, as far as I can see, is to provide care for the physical, mental and spiritual needs of the patient. And to help them come to terms with their illness, to accept the fact – which is a very hard fact to many people – that their life is going to end. I think that's sometimes even harder for the relatives. I suppose it's difficult to come to terms with the fact that someone they love is going to die. . . . It's to make the last remaining weeks or months or days as pleasant and as comfortable . . . as easy . . . for all parties as possible.

In this quotation we hear both the nurse's clear understanding of the principles of hospice care, and how she is beginning to transpose them into her own aims and ideals, and practice – that is helping the patient and, importantly, their family to come to terms with death while attempting to make the time remaining pleasant.

Cumulatively, the cluster of meanings associated with the word 'care' implied high standards and a personal, thoughtful, patient-centred approach. Teamwork was not an optional extra but vital to the principles of care. But the nurses' descriptions of care also tended to be imprecise, reflecting a universal difficulty in defining what 'care' means:

> Good care is being able to do as much as possible for a patient when they need it most. Some patients need a lot of help. And some don't need help, they just need someone to speak to.

> I think good care is getting near the person and really getting to know them.

... the type of caring you give one person wouldn't mean much to another.

They would describe it with reference to the skills it required such as 'listening', 'being there', 'being involved', 'spending time', 'doing the basics plus extra', but they also described it in terms of what it was not – a form of criticism of what nurses have sometimes been trained to do:

> She was a good nurse, but the patients didn't like her. You can over-nurse, you know.

> You can give them good care and be in a rush or rush them or tuck them in all tight. That's maybe doing all the proper things, but it's not good for the patient.

'Care' was used as an explanation for the purpose of the unit and a guiding principle against which standards of practice were measured. There is, of course, a problem associated with working to ideals because they are unachievable. As one dictionary notes, 'ideals are an image of perfection', but we are not perfect beings. With such high standards it is hard to get 'care' right, but easy to be inadequate:

> ... they need so much. Really so much attention, and when you canna give them it, it's really horrible. 'Cos you go off work feeling shattered, and feel you haven't done anything for them.

Analysis – two uses of 'care'

Accepting that the word 'care' was associated with a cluster of meanings, practical and analytic, it helps to specify two main themes in its use – one as principle and the second as an aspect of the labour of caring. In the quotations given above we can decipher both the nurses' ideals and the emotional energy used to work toward those ideals – that is emotional labour (James 1989).

The word 'labour' is used advisedly in association with emotion because of its sense of being hard, tiring, requiring some knowledge and understanding of what is to be done, together with the requisite organization and management. Though the emotional labour and its outcomes can rarely be seen or measured it has a considerable effect which is usually ignored in analysis, and which we are currently having difficulty accommodating within the workload measurement systems being developed (Smith 1991).

In nursing terms, emotional labour can be as exhausting as physical labour. Sitting with a distressed person, listening to someone when they are angry, depressed, resentful or sad, and acquiring the ability to be able to just 'be' with someone who is lonely, frightened or in pain, are highly taxing. Emotional labour is as demanding as physical labour. After a sustained time at either a nurse needs a rest or an alternative. Emotional labour requires learned skills in the same way that physical labour does, and recognition of this has led to the enormous growth of the 'human relationships' aspect of nurse education and training. But emotional labour also needs a form of organization and management different to the rigidity of the work ethic where principles of predictability and control dominate. 'Care' as emotional labour requires the flexibility to respond to different circumstances as they arise in ways that cannot be strictly timetabled but which nevertheless, have an internally coherent form of organization.

Thus 'care' is pragmatic as well as symbolic. As the nurses referred to it, 'care' included valued skills of attention, warmth, involvement and empathetic understanding, and techniques of assessment and intervention. This is highly significant where an 'individual patient care' service is being encouraged. It embodies an approach to understanding needs together with some practical means of achieving them. Nevertheless, 'care' usually remains invisible. No one knows it has been done, and it is exceedingly hard to estimate its value in quantitative terms and therefore to take adequate account of its practical effect.

Work

Observations

In contrast to 'care', 'work' was much more straightforward because for the most part 'work' was visible and could be timetabled. It is also the aspect of 'total work' which is easily imposed and for which staff are most accountable. Though 'work' involves 'tasks', as it was used at Byresfold the term meant more than the standard nursing 'task allocation' implies for it also included maintenance work, paper work, meetings, and escort duty. So although 'work' was often used in the common-sense meaning of paid labour ('I have to work, we need the money'), it was also used to describe the physical tasks associated with being at Byresfold. 'Work' could be described as structuring the day, and laying down a broad outline of patient and staff routines. As the Sister said:

> It's not really a question of its laid law. We're all open to ideas. But I really do feel that there are certain routines. I think you have to do that. But it's not a discipline that's inflexible.

One problem about doing 'work' is that the pressure to complete physical labours can dominate other elements of 'total care' and when the Byresfold staff were under pressure, physical work was carried out at the expense of spending time talking to frightened patients:

> Sometimes they want to speak to you. They so much want the time with you. And you're standing there, sorta about to say 'come on, I've got work

to do'. Because you've got so much other stuff to do, and they're so much just wanting to speak to you.

Though 'work' itself could be a cause of pressure, especially if there were staff shortages, the staff were precise about what they needed to do, and when it had come to an end:

> If you're really short, you go at such a rate. On lates, if there are 4 staff on, 2 do drugs. . . . Well that's alright if you've got someone who's been here for a while and can lift. But recently I've had a few lates with the new girls, and it's quite a strain. And I get all excited wondering if I'm going to get through the work.

One further point made in this last quotation is how the order of the Unit, indeed most would say the standards of caring work, is affected by staff famili-arity with the unit. Training new staff meant that not only had they to be initiated into the routines of the unit, but also Byresfold's philosophy, the types of assessment of patient need, and the difference of pace.

Though there are difficulties associated with 'work', the pressures to achieve it are of a different order to those associated with 'care'. 'Work' is physical activity, doing things. 'Work' is specifiable and time limited, and at Byresfold it could be seen to have been done. Through explanations of work, staff were able to define what was expected of them, and what to expect of themselves. So the finite and distinct demands of 'work' could be used as a protective barrier to regulate and counterbalance the seemingly endless demands of 'care' for, as an auxiliary pointed out, without the physical part, the emotional part of the work would have been overwhelming.

Analysis – physical labour and paid labour

In terms of priorities in 'total work', the mental timetables of 'work to be done' shaped the day and work was a key measure of a nurse's familiarity with Byresfold. The skills involved in the physical labour included assessment of what was needed, the ability to carry it out and the competent organizing of priorities to the optimum satisfaction of patients, staff and the hospice as a whole. In this sense 'work' is similar to 'care' because it has practical and symbolic value but, being visible and accountable, it becomes central to the organization of 'caring work' unless formal and specific measures are taken to ensure that it does not dominate. 'Emotional labour' at Byresfold had no formal place except as an integral part of the physical labour, and the schedules around which the work was organized.

The balance of care to work can therefore be used as a measure of the order of priorities in a unit, but also of dissonance. Nurses notably felt most uncertain of their role and abilities when the tensions between the work to be done and their caring aspirations were most obvious.

'Work' in terms of paid employment was as significant as physical labour. The parameters of paid work, the shifts, variations in pay, and different training and education, curtail one of the tyrannies of care – the never achievable quest for perfect 'care' for all patients. Work then, is also a reference to formal and informal management structures which control who gives patient care and when.

Reading through the taped conversations it became clear that systems of professional status structure the working relations and the 'work'. These organizational influences had their effect inter-professionally as well as intra-professionally so that auxiliaries hesitated before initiating a conversation with the doctors. In contrast the newly appointed staff nurses sought the doctors' company for a chat as much as for an exchange of information, as if they were establishing their new status as 'trained staff' by such proximity.

It is easy to imply that 'work' is the villain of the piece. I would argue that on the contrary it is what makes 'care' possible. It enabled the nurses to retain the vision and their aspirations while allowing them to set mental boundaries on what they could reasonably expect of themselves. 'Work' thereby served a vital purpose in slowing down 'battle-fatigue' or burnout (Maslach 1982; Earnshaw-Smith 1987; Vachon 1987). The key importance of 'care' to 'work' therefore is balance, but lest we become complacent over how effective we are in achieving the balance, it is worth remembering a recent report of degradation of the elderly through what could be analysed as a pure 'work' orientation (Counsel and Care 1991).

Carework

Observations

And so we come to what I refer to as 'carework'. One use of 'carework' is as an analysis of the art of the possible, the ideals and the emotional labour intertwined with the imposed constraints of physical labour. Carework is a recognition of the negotiable tension between the principles and the skills involved in giving personal attention to individual patients and the routinization necessary in any organization (Silverman 1970; Salaman 1979; Thompson 1983).

At an applied level carework is best illustrated through an example – one that came from fieldwork at the first hospice. A patient was thought to be on the point of dying and was due to be turned. However it was right at the end of the shift and the staff decided to leave the 'turning' for the next shift. This was because they did not want to precipitate the death by the turning, and then be put in the position of feeling obliged to carry out 'last offices' making them very late off the shift. Such a decision was not made without concern for the patient, since the next shift were informed as soon as they arrived, so the patient would not have suffered. On the other hand it also took account of the staff's desire to leave on time. It was not insensitive, but it was an agreed form of adjusting the good of the patient to the parameters of work.

Another example of 'carework' which came from the second hospice was the way in which predictions of death were used (usually unconsciously) both in a 'caring' sense – planning for the ideal of a 'dignified death', and also as a means of planning workload. Using 'predictions' families could be helped to decide whether to come to the unit or not, and families and staff were helped to anticipate the sorrow of their loss. Also, though to a lesser extent, predictions helped the staff plan their 'work', for death brings with it a series of time-consuming physical tasks.

There were numerous other illustrations of 'carework', including how the idealized perspective of a 'family unit' (a domestic analogy) was balanced against that of 'teamwork' (a workplace reference) (James 1988), and the way in which the aspirations and practices of 'normal death' developed (James 1986). In all instances, 'carework' was a means by which staff could take account of factors over which they felt they had minimal influence, and which often, though not always, involved hierarchical decision-making.

Analysis

'Carework' can be used for two purposes, one descriptive, one analytic. Its descriptive form is not static but shows nursing practices to be the product of the ambiguities and interests with which both 'care' and 'work' are invested. Importantly it allowed the staff an informal means of evaluating their practice against their ideals. By using 'work' with all its ramifications as a means of explaining the constraints on their 'care' they were able to preserve their vision of their principles, whilst accepting the limitations of their practice. I would argue that this was an important function, for when an individual's vision of their service is lost, there is little to strive for and compromise becomes too easy.

In its second, analytic form, carework can be used as a means of connecting together two frequently distinct frameworks with separate social histories which are joined together in a wide range of circumstances as 'caring work'. Looking at the connections between the domestic, private, women's domain of 'care' and the public, paid, male-dominated arena of 'work' helps us to examine structural restraints on radical development.

Though initially carework was used to understand the relationship between care and work in one hospice unit at a specific historical moment, the difficulties exposed are common to nurses' in a wide variety of circumstances (Nethercott 1991; Turnock 1991). The ways in which these difficulties, or tensions, between 'care' and 'work' become obvious vary with different circumstances but, for the most part, the underlying causes do not. By attempting to compare and contrast the 'work' and 'domestic care' frameworks, we can deconstruct and examine the 'tensions' whether they are at unit or policy levels.

An example of difficulties at unit level is provided by Davies who points out that work routines protect the nurse 'on the one hand from dealing with the emotional strain of continually working through new interactions with the patient, and on the other from the strain of having to negotiate from a position of weakness, with the doctor' (Davies 1977: 491). Thus routines are a product of working relations and conditions as well as the emotional labour of making relationships – a compromise on 'patient-centred care' certainly, but one based on sound reasoning.

At an organizational level bringing together the domestic and work ideologies helps us to understand why, as Rowbotham (1973) noted, 'sentiment' and 'emotion' have not generally been deemed a suitable part of 'work' (James 1989). Economic and efficiency criteria shape the caring services, and 'total care' costs money, as does any identification of need and demand (*Lancet* 1988). Visions of care require political will, the passage of time and, whatever the rhetoric, the resources to put ideals into practice.

> The problem is that nominal powers are useless unless there is the money, the authority and the will to use them. Despite its importance, nursing has always been subordinate in the NHS and has failed to claim or win the sources it needs.
>
> (Salvage 1985: 55)

While the workplace orientation of the biomedical emphasis on body malfunction prescribes the kind of health care services deemed appropriate for cure, despite post-war developments there is still considerable circumspection about the domestic type of knowledge which demands more 'care'.

Synthesis – a comment

In organizational terms in recent years nurses have set a mammoth task. Principles of 'total care', 'individual patient care', 'holistic care' and of developing multidisciplinary teamwork are being developed within a bureaucratic health care system with a long history of division. Yet these 'care' principles need to emerge in forms in which they can be sustained despite economic and political change. For this reason the ways in which principles of 'care' are adapted into practice within the workplace become central to questions of whether nursing can achieve its aspirations. Policy-makers therefore become intermediaries – a vital influence on the ways in which principles are translated into action plans before they are adopted in clinical practice.

Using the sociology of organization and of work as a theoretical underpinning, I have suggested that the division between care, work and carework can be used in several ways. In conclusion I raise the question of whether we should be developing our nursing knowledge and policies on the basis of synthesis (carework), or whether thesis (care) and antithesis (work) should remain.

Using carework helps us to understand the gaps between the ideals and practice, the relation of the individual to the organization, and the demands of emotional labour relative to physical labour. I suggest that, analytically, it is vital that the concepts remain antagonistically separate – as thesis and antithesis suggest they should. Within this format 'carework' can serve as a critique of the way nursing outcomes are conceptualized, for using concepts of care and work as protagonists can highlight political, economic, social and professional interests which vie for power within health care systems. Divisions between 'care' and 'work' mean that neither is accepted at face value. Instead they are constantly referred back to their roots in motivation, principle, policy and practice.

An alternative, or complementary use of care, work and carework is as a pragmatic, non-judgemental synthesis, a way of coming to terms with the daily organizational constraints on what can be achieved within workplace care. In my own (highly intermittent) practice, I use care, work and carework as a quick measure – what are the aims of the ward/unit; what constraints do the staff work within, and how does compromise or adaptation emerge in practice? This system accepts that as health practitioners, entirely appropriately, we have ideals, visions of patient care, which are beyond immediate reach. It also accepts the inevitable gap between these ideals and workplace demands and without being in despair at having failed to achieve them, encourages us to question what causes the gaps in order to be able to deal with them more effectively and improve the quality of 'carework'.

Current emphasis on the 'quality of care' in health services poses many challenges as we attempt to convey the essence of nursing's contribution to health outcomes. In these circumstances the use of 'carework' as a conceptual tool can help broaden our thinking and our understanding. What are the constraints of 'workplace' relative to 'domestic care'? Where do the similarities and differences lie, and where should the differences lie?

9

Nursing policy, the supply and demand for nurses: Towards a clinical career structure for nurses

Dirk Keyzer

Writing from the perspective of a nurse civil servant, Dirk Keyzer examines the relationship between nursing policy, changing definitions of nursing and labour market fluctuations. He sees the introduction of the clinical pay structure and the development of related vocational educational programmes as valid attempts to develop practice policies in response to a number of changes in the organization of nursing such as the shift away from a hierarchical bureaucracy towards a meritocracy; the introduction of manager-led rather than profession-led organization; and the rise of the clinical nurse. Despite the initial and perhaps inevitable teething problems with the clinical grading review, Dirk Keyzer sees the rise of the clinical career as the logical answer to the need to value clinical nursing skills and to establish the professional career in an appropriate juxtaposition with general management and with medicine.

Disclaimer

The following chapter has been cleared with the Welsh Office and approval has been given subject to the following disclaimer:

The opinions expressed in this chapter are those of the author, based on published research and current nursing literature, utilizing a specific theoretical framework for analysis. These personal opinions do not reflect those of the Secretary of State for Wales, nor should they be viewed as carrying any implications for official Welsh Office policy.

Introduction

This chapter presents and discusses some issues facing the nursing profession in a changing social and organizational climate. The issues confronting nursing arise from:

1 The demographic trends and the effect these will have on the labour market.
2 The moves towards a management-led organization, and the replacement of the bureaucracy associated with the Salmon Report (MoH, SHHD 1966) by a meritocracy.
3 The greater emphasis on progressional vocational education during and after secondary education and the implications for nursing education.
4 Future developments in manpower planning.

These issues set the scene in which future nursing policies and strategies will be formed and failure to tackle them could result in the demise of the profession.

Nursing policy is defined here as the actions nurse leaders take to promote, maintain and secure professional boundaries in pursuit of two main goals: to provide a service to the client and to secure the profession's survival in a changing organizational and social climate.

Nursing and the labour market

The fortunes of nursing and the policies adopted by the profession are directly linked to the ups and downs of the female labour market. Even though the NHS has been able to train more nurses than it required in the past, changes in the job opportunities for women have had and will continue to have, an impact on the recruitment and retention of nurses. The UKCC's suggested reforms of nurse education draw attention to the reduction of nursing's traditional labour pool, young female school leavers, and the NHS's position in an increasingly competitive labour market (UKCC 1986a).

The Project 2000 proposals' emphasis on a practitioner role for one level of registered nurse appears to be signalling a change in the profession's conception of the role of the nurse (UKCC 1986a). There is a strong contrast with the recommendations of the Salmon Report (MoH, SHHD 1966), which had finally established an hierarchical bureaucracy giving nursing an equal voice in the decision-making process on a par with doctors and administrators. That consolidation of the profession's powerbase in the management structure of the NHS signified the achievement of a long-term nursing occupational strategy, originating in the Nightingale hospitals of the mid and late nineteenth century. However, although the period between the Salmon Report and its review by Griffiths (DHSS 1983), witnessed the consolidation of nursing power in the organizational role of the nurse manager, this organizational power was bought at the expense of the professional, that is practitioner, role of the registered nurse. The practitioner role was further debased by the handing over of direct care-giving activities to a second level of registered nurse, student nurses and nursing auxiliaries, and the incorporation of these nursing organizational policies into the personnel planning strategies for the NHS (Keyzer 1988).

The introduction of general management following the Griffiths Report has all but obliterated the hierarchical bureaucracy created by the Salmon Report. Nursing must now face the reality that past professional strategies have denied it the power base in clinical practice it now requires to promote leaders who will remain in nursing practice and to have its voice heard in the clinical decision-making process. Past strategies will no longer serve us well in this new environment. How then can we enable our colleagues to revise their attitudes towards the previously debased clinical role of the nurse? The attitudinal changes required to promote the practitioner role for the clinical nurse depend on planned educational programmes and the management of change within the clinical environment. Such attitudinal changes are necessary not only in nurses but also in the diverse occupational groups whose roles and work overlap with that of the nurse.

Managerialism: a threat to nursing boundaries?

It is uncertain whether or not the nursing profession foresaw the advent of general managers and, in view of this, decided to adjust its policies towards the practitioner role for the registered nurse. What is certain is that the challenge to the traditional nursing power structures posed by the introduction of general management, occurred at a point in time before the profession had time to consolidate its new concepts of a practitioner nurse. Thus, the shift in organizational power, from the nurse manager towards the general manager, appeared to throw some of the members of the nursing profession into disarray. The outward appearance was of a profession suddenly confronted with a situation in which it had to defend its boundaries, at all levels of the organization, against a new and powerful organizational group, general managers. Without a practitioner role for the registered nurse, with its attendant powerbase in the clinical areas, it must have appeared to some nurses that they would no longer be able to control their education and practice.

The nursing profession will have to acknowledge that as a major organizational power general managers have the authority to define nursing; to create new divisions of labour within the health care team; and to re-think nursing's place within the new order. This is manifest in the new clinical grading structure negotiated between the Management and Staff Sides of the Nursing and Midwifery Staffs Negotiation Council, and introduced in 1988 (DHSS 1988). The intent behind this new pay structure was to acknowledge the clinical expertise and responsibilities held by clinical nurses. The creation of this new pay scale has to be viewed as a radical change in the culture of the traditional nursing organization, not least because it has provided a measure of the worth managers give to the work allocated to different grades of nurse. In an organization that has previously kept the roles and work of qualified and unqualified nurses so interchangeable that nursing auxiliaries, student nurses and registered nurses carry out the same care giving activities, any differentiation between the categories of nurse is a significant break with the past. No longer can individual members of the profession stand still, safe in the knowledge that length of service alone will waft them upwards to district and regional executive nursing posts. Competition, education and demonstrated expertise are now the order of the day for those seeking advancement in health care organizations.

A clinical career structure is based on the premise that it will provide tangible evidence of the value general managers place on the work of clinical nurses. This premise presents a considerable challenge to an organization which has always placed a greater value on the managerial than the clinical role of the nurse. The new clinical career structure must be based on the following beliefs:

1 That nurses are paid according to their ability to perform a given job as defined by a specific job description differentiating clinical competencies.
2 That a given nursing job is worth only so much and that there is a maximum level of pay for that job.
3 That length of service or seniority alone will not be rewarded in isolation from performance.
4 That nurses develop clinical expertise in specific clinical specialities through advanced education.
5 That expert nurses can integrate education and research into their daily practice.

A clinical career structure, therefore, introduces a meritocracy in line with the principles of general management. Nurses seeking career advancement through a clinical career structure will have to take on the appropriate level of responsibility and accountability for decision-making in relation to client care and resource management. A clinical career structure, supporting the practitioner role for the nurse, is a major challenge to the traditional nursing organization but one that must be met if nursing is to achieve its survival and service goals.

Education

The new clinical career ladder will also have important implications for the contents of the pre- and post-registration education programmes. The direct linkage between the structure of the organization and nursing career pathways will be reflected in the curriculum and discipline models presented to the students. In the past, the discrepancy between the curriculum model, representing the clinical role of the nurse, and the discipline model, supporting the managerial role of the nurse, was the main source of the dichotomy between theory and practice in nursing. This dichotomy may well persist if the profession's definition of nursing differs from that of the general manager. The definition of nursing held by the general manager in the future health care organization will dictate what is considered to be *bona fide* nursing knowledge in the clinical area and the classroom. In this way the distribution of power and the principles of social control in the clinical area will be reflected in the curriculum presented to the student. This course of events will have serious implications for nursing and its claims to professional status. How do the current reforms in nurse education appear in the light of these developments? Project 2000 is a far-reaching reform of nurse education, but it must be viewed in its wider social setting. Current government education policy has placed a greater emphasis on vocational training in the curriculum of the secondary education programme. This emphasis arises out of concerns expressed by industry over the skill mix present in its workforce. The 14–19 curriculum has undergone dramatic changes both in structure and types of qualifications since 1979. The introduction of new schemes BTEC, YTS, TVEI and NCVQ, amongst others, indicate the scale of innovation and the change towards progressional education programmes.

The term 'progression' has become increasingly popular in attempting to evaluate and establish relationships between different training initiatives and qualifications. It refers to the opportunity for students to progress into and between qualifications and for continuity of learning. Progression between qualifications also involves movement between different types of organizations which have their own cultures and values whether these be colleges of nursing, further education colleges, higher education establishments, or the workplace.

The new nurse education programme proposed in Project 2000 must be seen in the context of this progression. In particular, it must be viewed in the context of the four major areas of discussion about progression and policy-making associated with 14–19 training and education:

1 progression between 14–16 and 16–19 frameworks;
2 progression at 16+;
3 progression between levels of sector vocational qualifications;
4 success for adult returners to education and training.

The place of Project 2000 in this progression is central to future nurse recruitment and retention. The question of support workers, their numbers and levels are a part of the debate on progression and vocational education. Given the past misuse and abuse of untrained and registered nurses by the organization, including nurse managers, exemplified in the outcomes identified during the process of implementing the clinical grading review, can we justify the existence of 1st level registered nurses at the bedside? If patient services can be run on the inputs of so many nurses working out of grade, without any outward ill effect on patient outcomes, do we really need expensive education programmes such as that envisaged by Project 2000? This issue will have to be addressed if professional nursing is to survive.

Furthermore, we must ask ourselves if the statutory bodies' entry requirements and examinations are helpful in providing the flexible 'knowledgeable doer' promised by Project 2000, or merely barriers to obstruct the implementation of the general managers' plans for the organization?

Manpower planning

These questions lead into the issues associated with resource management. Nursing, as the largest single occupational group within health care organizations, is a vital resource. The management and utilization of this resource has direct implications for the care received by the client and the service offered by the profession to the organization and its subdivisions. The most simple definition of manpower planning is that it is a process whereby we ensure that the right people are in the right place at the right time. Even this simplistic definition suggests that manpower planning is more than just numbers and dependent on the knowledge and skills held by individuals which, in turn, are dependent on the education programmes available. Manpower planning includes the need to judge the appropriate skill mix required to provide health care. In considering the issues surrounding skill mix we must look at the knowledge and skills within the nursing service; how these relate to and complement the skills of other occupational groups; and nursing's boundaries with other occupational groups.

Manpower planning relies on accurate surveys of the external and internal labour pools. Demographic trends indicate that the external labour pool is shrinking. Thus nursing can no longer rely on a constant supply of female school leavers. As female labour becomes a comparative rarity in a competitive labour market, its value will increase. The sheer size of the nursing workforce makes any increase in cost a serious consideration in providing health care. The increased cost of employing large numbers of female workers may have one of two contrasting effects on the future of nursing:

1 The increased cost will upgrade the status of nursing as a profession.
2 The increased cost will demand the opening up of nursing practice to ensure the constant supply of 'pairs of hands' at affordable costs.

To offset this reduction in their traditional labour pool both the UKKC (1986a) and the managers of the service have suggested a widening of the entry gate to professional nurse education and the recruitment of mature men and women to the new nurse education programmes. At the time of writing there is also considerable work being carried out by the National Health Service Training Agency (NHSTA), to ensure that future health care assistants will have the training to enable them to carry out the work expected of them by the managers of the service. There is, however, evidence to suggest a secularly expanding labour market for part-time female workers outside the NHS. Thus the assumption that the deficits in nurse learner recruitment can be offset by recruiting more mature female workers into nursing may have been ill-founded.

Similarly, there is little evidence to support the assumption that nursing will attract more young and mature men into the service. Nurse recruitment, therefore, may be confined to the traditional labour pool in an increasingly competitive labour market. Consequently the role of personnel management assumes a vital importance in retaining existing nurse personnel in order to maintain existing stocks of qualified and unqualified nurses. General managers must formulate recruitment and retention strategies that provide lateral and vertical professional development within the chosen field of practice, and that meet the professional and social needs of married and unmarried men and women and that are on a par with those educational, health and welfare pro-grammes offered by industries outside the NHS. Moreover, the skills held by clinical nurses will have to be organized into a clinical career structure which differentiates the levels of skills held and decisions taken by clinical nurses in the hospital and community settings.

Conclusions

The historical development of the nursing profession in the UK indicates that the profession will have to adjust its traditional strategies to suit the prevailing social climate. The problems facing general managers today, and in the near future, are different from those of the past. The imbalance between the supply and demand for nurses stems from the decrease in the numbers of young men and women entering the labour market and the reduction in the nursing profession's traditional labour pool. The mismatch between the supply and demand for both male and female workers, across all sections of the labour market, will require a reorganization of work practices and a revision of the gender division of labour in the home and the work place. General managers and members of the nursing profession will have to change their perceptions of nurses and nursing work, and reassess the impact that family life and family size have on the recruitment and retention of male and female nurses.

In the past nurses looked to their nurse managers for leadership. The intro-duction of general managers appears to have removed that focus of professional leadership. In the future, nurses will have to identify new leaders. They may be found in the clinical areas of the NHS. They may also be found in academic establishments for the increasing access to higher education for nurses in the 1970s, particularly the setting up of academic departments of nursing, has resulted in a steady stream of research reports demanding change in traditional nurse education programmes and policy on the role of the nurse.

It seems clear, however, that simply to retreat behind professional barriers and to wait for a hero innovator to come along to solve these problems could have catastrophic results for the profession as we know it and the service offered to the public. Thus the options can be stated starkly:

1 The profession takes on the management of change and meets the challenge of that change; or
2 the profession negates its responsibilities to manage the change and gives those responsibilities over to other occupational groups.

The choices are simple: the survival and growth of nursing, or its demise.

Acknowledgements

The writer acknowledges the support given by Miss M. Bull, Chief Nursing Officer, Welsh Office; and Mr A. Beattie, Head of Department of Health and Welfare Studies, London University Institute of Education, in the preparation and presentation of this chapter.

References

Abbott, A. (1988). *The System of Professions: An Essay on the Division of Expert Labour.* University of Chicago Press.

Abel-Smith, B. (1960). *A History of the Nursing Profession.* London, Heinemann.

Abercrombie, N. *et al.* (1984). *The Penguin Dictionary of Sociology.* Harmondsworth, Penguin.

American Medical Association (1989). *Philosophy, Structure and Content of the Curriculum for the Registered Care Technician.* Chicago, American Medical Association.

Arber, S. and Gilbert, N. (1989). 'Men: the forgotten carers', *Sociology* **23**, 1, 111–18.

Armstrong, D. (1983a). 'The fabrication of nurse–patient relationships', *Social Science and Medicine* **17**, 8, 457–60.

Armstrong, D. (1983b). *Political Anatomy of the Body.* Cambridge University Press.

Arney, W. and Bergen, B. (1983). 'The anomaly, the chronic patient and the play of medical power', *Sociology of Health and Illness* **5**, 1, 11–24.

Astill, J. L. and Watkin, D. F. L. (1987). 'What does a house-surgeon on call for the wards do?', *Lancet* **i**, 1363–5.

Atkinson, J. (1986). *Changing Working Patterns: How Companies Achieve Flexibility to Meet New Needs.* Institute of Manpower Studies, National Economic Development Office.

Austin, R. (1977). 'Sex and gender: the future of nursing', *Nursing Times* 25 August, Occasional Paper, **73**, 34, 113–16.

Bain, P. G. *et al.* (1990). 'Workload of preregistration house officers', *British Medical Journal* **300**, 1463.

Baxter, C. (1987). *The Black Nurse: An Endangered Species.* Training in Health and Race, National Extension College.

Beecham, L. (1990). 'Reservations on nurse prescribing', *British Medical Journal* **300**, 1275–6.

Bellaby, P. and Oribabor, P. (1980). 'The history of the present: contradiction and struggle in nursing', in C. Davies (ed.) *Rewriting Nursing History*. London, Croom Helm.

Bevan, S. *et al.* (1990). *Women in Hospital Pharmacy*. IMS Report No. 182, Brighton, Institute of Manpower Studies.

Blunden, R. and Kushlick, A. (1974). *Research and the Care of Elderly People*. Research Report 110, Winchester, Health Care Evaluation Team.

Bond, S. *et al.* (1990). *Primary Nursing and Primary Medical Care: A Comparative Study in Community Hospitals*. Health Care Research Unit Report No. 39, University of Newcastle upon Tyne School of Health Care Sciences.

Bosanquet, N. and Gerard, K. (1985). *Nursing Manpower: Recent Trends and Policy Options*. Discussion Paper 9, Centre for Health Economics, University of York.

Branham, J. (1982). *Practical Manpower Planning*. London, Institute of Personnel Management.

Briggs, A. (1972). *Committee on Nursing*. Cmnd. 5115, London, HMSO.

Bright, J. (1985). *A Critique of Methods for Determining Nurse Staffing Levels in Hospitals*. DHSS Operational Research Service, London, DHSS.

Brittain, V. (1984). *Testament of Youth*. London, Virago.

Brocklehurst, J. and Andrews, K. (1987). 'Nurse staffing in geriatric wards', *Nursing Times* 4 February, 48–51.

Brook, E. and Davis, A. (eds) (1985). *Women, the Family and Social Work*. London, Tavistock.

Brown, R. G. S. (1975). 'Male nurses' careers', *Nursing Times* 25 September, 71, 39, 97–9.

Buchan, J. (1987). 'A shared future', *Nursing Times* 28 January, 83, 4, 44–5.

Buchan, J. (1990a). 'Coming and going', *Nursing Standard* 3 January, 4, 15, 47–9.

Buchan, J. (1990b). 'Growing independents', *Nursing Standard* 28 March, 4, 27, 48.

Buchan, J. (1990c). 'Breaking Away', *Nursing Times* 17 October, 86, 42, 20.

Buchan, J. *et al.* (1989). *Grade Expectations: Clinical Grading and Nurse Mobility*. IMS Report No. 176, Brighton, Institute of Manpower Studies.

Bucher, R. and Strauss, A. L. (1961). 'Professions in Process', *American Journal of Sociology* 66, 325–34.

Buckenham, J. and McGrath, G. (1983). *The Social Reality of Nursing*. Balgowlah, Australia, ADIS Health Science Press.

Bytheway, W. (1987). 'Male carers: questions of intervention', in conference proceedings ed. J. Twigg from *Evaluating Carer Support*. York, Social Policy Research Unit.

Calnan, M. (1987). *Health and Illness: The Lay Perspective*. London, Tavistock.

Carling, E. (1930). 'Recruitment for Nursing', *Lancet* 11 October, 826.

Carpenter, M. (1977). 'The new managerialism and professionalism in nursing', in M. Stacey, M. Reid and C. Heath (eds) *Health and the Division of Labour*. Beckenham, Croom Helm.

Central Health Services Council (1966). *The Post-Certificate Training and Education of Nurses: a Report by a Sub-committee of the Standing Nurse Advisory Committee*. (Chairman, Miss Muriel Powell), London, HMSO.

Central Statistical Office (1991). *Social Trends*. London, CSO.

Centre for Health and Social Research (1990). *The Limbo Project*. Ulster, University of Ulster.

Chapman, C. (1985). *Theory of Nursing: Practical Application*. London, Harper & Row.

Clay, T. (1986). 'Where have all the women gone?', *Lampada* Spring, 7, 20–2.

Clay, T. (1987). *Nurses: Power and Politics*. London, Heinemann.

Cockayne, E. (1988). Interview by A. M. Rafferty with Dame Elizabeth Cockayne.

Counsel and Care (1991). *Not Such Private Places*. Twyman House, 16 Bonny Street, London.

Daily Express (1937). 'Nursing romance: nurses who lose it by long hours', 18 November.

Daily Sketch (1937a). 'Nurses of Britain plan their case', 2 November.

Daily Sketch (1937b). 'Dragooned by petty rules: nurses ask for humane treatment', 9 November.

Dalley, G. (1988). *Ideologies of Caring: Rethinking Community and Collectivism*. London, Macmillan.

Davies, C. (1976). 'Experience of dependency and control in work: the case of nurses', *Journal of Advanced Nursing* 1, 1, 273–82.

Davies, C. (1977). 'Continuities in the development of hospital nursing in Britain', *Journal of Advanced Nursing* 1, 2, 479–93.

Davies, C. (ed.) (1980). *Rewriting Nursing History*. London, Croom Helm.

Davies, C. (1990). *The Collapse of the Conventional Career*. London, English National Board.

Davies, C. and Rosser, J. (1986). *Processes of Discrimination: a Study of Women Working in the NHS*. DHSS, London, HMSO.

Delamothe, T. (1988). 'Not a profession, not a career', *British Medical Journal* 296, 271–4.

Department of Employment (1989). *New Earnings Survey*. London, HMSO.

Department of Health (1989a). *A Strategy for Nursing*. Report of the Steering Group, Nursing Division, London, DoH.

Department of Health (1989b). *Report of the Advisory Group on Nurse Prescribing*. London, DoH.

Department of Health (1989c). *The Extending Role of the Nurse*. Report of a Working Party, (PL/CMO (89)7 and 10), London, Health Publications Unit, DoH.

Department of Health (1990a). *Health and Personal Social Services for England*. London, HMSO.

Department of Health (1990b). *NHS Workforce in England* 1990 Edition. London, HMSO.

Department of Health and Social Security – Management Services (NHS) (1971). *Organisation of the Junior Hospital Doctors*. London, HMSO.

Department of Health and Social Security (1972). *Management Arrangements for the Reorganized National Health Service*. London, HMSO.

Department of Health and Social Security (1976). *Sharing Resources for Health in England*. Report of the Resource Allocation Working Party, London, HMSO.

Department of Health and Social Security (1977). *The Extending Role of the Clinical Nurse – Legal Implications and Training Requirements*. HC(77)22, London, DHSS.

Department of Health and Social Security (1983). *NHS Management Inquiry (The Griffiths Report)*. DNA (83)38, London, DHSS.

Department of Health and Social Security (1984). *Health Service Management: Implementation of the NHS Management Inquiry Report*. HC(84)13, London, DHSS.

Department of Health and Social Security (1986a). *Neighbourhood Nursing: a Focus for Care*. Report of the Community Nursing Review in England (Chairman, Julia Cumberlege), London, HMSO.

Department of Health and Social Security (1986b). *Hospital Medical Staffing: Achieving a Balance*. London, HMSO.

Department of Health and Social Security (1988). 'Review body for nursing staff, midwives, health visitors and the professions allied to medicine', *Fifth Report on Nursing Staff, Midwives and Health Visitors*. (Chairman, Sir James Cleminson), Cmnd 360, London, HMSO.

Department of Health and Social Security, Scottish Home and Health Department, Welsh Office (1969). *Report on Working Party on Management Structures in the Local Authority Nursing Services*. (Chairman, E.L. Mayston), London, DHSS.

Department of Health and Social Security and Welsh Office (1979). *Patients First: Consultative Paper on the Structure and Management of the NHS in England and Wales*. London, HMSO.

Department of Health, Department of Social Security, Welsh Office and Scottish Office (1989a). *Caring for People*. Cmnd. 849, London, HMSO.

Department of Health, Scottish Home and Health Department, Welsh Office and Northern Ireland Office (1989b). *Working for Patients*. Cmnd. 555, London, HMSO.

Dex, S. (1985). *The Sexual Division of Work*. Brighton, Wheatsheaf.

Dingwall, R. (1972). 'Nursing: towards a male dominated profession', *Nursing Times* 12 October, **68**, 41, 1294–5.

Dingwall, R. (1979). 'The place of men in nursing', in M. Colledge and D. Jones (eds) *Readings in Nursing*. Edinburgh, Churchill Livingstone.

Dingwall, R. *et al.* (1988). *An Introduction to the Social History of Nursing*. London, Routledge.

Donnison, J. (1977). *Midwives and Medical Men: A History of Inter-Professional Rivalries and Women's Rights*. London, Heinemann.

Doyal, L. (1979). *The Political Economy of Health*. London, Pluto.

Earnshaw-Smith, E. (1987). 'We don't need to be God after all', *Palliative Medicine* 1, 2, 154–61.

Eldridge, J. (1980). *Recent British Sociology*. London, Macmillan.

Feminist Review (1988). Special volume on child abuse, January.

Fitzgerald, M. (1990). Personal communication with Kate Robinson (author of Chapter 2).

Flynn, N. (1990). *Public Sector Management*. Hertfordshire, Harvester Wheatsheaf.

Foucault, M. (1976). *The Birth of the Clinic*. London, Tavistock.

Freidson, E. (1970). *Profession of Medicine: A Study of the Sociology of Applied Knowledge*. New York, Dodd Mead.

Gamarnikow, E. (1978). 'Sexual division of labour: the case of nursing', in A. Wolpe and A. Huhn (eds) *Feminism and Materialism*. London, Routledge Kegan Paul.

Giovanetti, P. (1986). 'Evaluation of primary nursing', in *Annual Review of Nursing Research* 4, 127–51.

Gordon, P. (1988). *Race in Britain: A Research and Information Guide*. Runnymede Trust.

Graham, H. (1983). 'Caring: a labour of love', in J. Finch and D. Groves (eds) *A Labour of Love*. London, Routledge & Kegan Paul.

Graham, H. (1991). 'The concept of caring in feminist research: the case of domestic service', *Sociology* 25, 1, 61–78.

Gray, A. (1986). 'Anatomy of a profession', *Nursing Times* 26 March, **82**, 13, 24–6.

Gray, A. (1987). *The Economics of Nursing: A Literature Review*. Nursing Policy Studies 2, NPSC, University of Warwick.

Gray, A. (1989). 'The NHS and the history of nurses' pay', *History of Nursing Bulletin* 2, 8, 15–29.

Green, J. *et al.* (1986). *The Division of Labour. Child Care and Development Group.* University of Cambridge.

Habermas, J. (1976). *Legitimation Crisis.* London, Heinemann.

Hammersley, M. and Atkinson, P. (1983). *Ethnography: Principles in Practice.* London, Tavistock.

Hearn, J. and Parkin, W. (1987). *Sex at Work.* Brighton, Wheatsheaf.

Heclo, H. (1972). 'Review article: policy analysis', *British Journal of Political Science* 2, 83–108.

Held, D. (1989). *Political Theory and the Modern State: Essays on State, Power and Democracy.* Cambridge, Polity.

Henderson, G. (1990). 'Nurse role issue must be resolved', *Hospital Doctor* 4 January, 7.

Henderson, V. (1966). *The Nature of Nursing.* London, Collier-McMillan.

Hicks, C. (1982). 'Racism in nursing', *Nursing Times* 12 May, 78, 18, 789–91.

Hockey, L. (1976). *Women in Nursing.* London, Hodder & Stoughton.

Hockey, L. (1979). 'The role of the nurse', in D. Doyle (ed.) *Terminal Care.* Edinburgh, Churchill Livingstone.

Holland, J. (1980). *Women and Work.* Bedford Way Papers, No. 6, London, Heinemann.

House of Commons (1926). *Report of the Select Committee on the General Nursing Council.* London, HMSO.

Hutt, R. *et al.* (1985). *The Manpower Implications of Possible Changes in Basic Nurse Training.* A Report to the RCN's Commission on Nursing Education, London, RCN.

Hutter, B. and Williams, G. (eds) (1981). *Controlling Women: the Normal and the Deviant.* London, Croom Helm.

Iglehart, J. K. (1987). 'Problems facing the nursing profession', *New England Journal of Medicine* 317, 646–51.

James, V. (1986). 'Care and work in nursing the dying', unpublished PhD thesis, University of Aberdeen.

James, V. (1988). 'A family and a team', in A. Gilmore and S. Gilmore (eds) *A Safer Way of Death.* New York, Plenum.

James, V. (1989). 'Emotional labour', *Sociological Review* 37, 1, 15–42.

Johns, C. (1989). 'The impact of introducing primary nursing on the culture of a community hospital', unpublished MSc dissertation, Cardiff, University of Wales.

Keyzer, D. M. (1988). 'Challenging role boundaries: conceptual frameworks for understanding the conflict arising from the implementation of the nursing process in practice', in R. White (ed.) *Political Issues in Nursing: Past, Present and Future.* Vol. 3, pp. 95–119, Chichester, Wiley.

Kirschling, J. (1986). 'The experience of terminal illness on adult family members', *Hospice Journal* 12, 1, 121–38.

Klein, R. (1983). *The Politics of the National Health Service.* London, Longman.

Lancet (1931a). 'The Lancet Commission on Nursing', first interim report, 28 February, 451–6.

Lancet (1931b). 'The Lancet Commission on Nursing', second interim report, Special Supplement, 15 August, i–xxiv.

Lancet (1932). *The Lancet Commission on Nursing.* Final Report.

Lancet (1933). 'The Lancet Commission on Nursing', 18 February, 369–70.

Lancet (1988). 'Medical care of newborn babies', 10 December, 1344–6.

Lancet (1990). 'A suitable case for intimacy', **336**, 217–18.

Lathlean, J. (1987). *Job Sharing a Ward Sister's Post*. London, Riverside Health Authority.

Law Harrison, L. (1990). 'Maintaining the ethic of caring in nursing', *Journal of Advanced Nursing* **15**, 2, 125–7.

Lee, M. E. (1979). 'Towards better care: "primary nursing"'. *Nursing Times* Occasional Paper, 20/27 December, **75**, 33, 133–5.

Leeson, J. and Gray, J. (1978). *Women and Medicine*. London, Tavistock.

Leininger, M. (1984). *Care: The Essence of Nursing and Health*. New Jersey, Slack Inc.

MacGuire, J. (1980). 'Nursing: none is held in higher esteem . . . Occupational control and the position of women in nursing', in R. Silverstone and A. Ward (eds) *Careers of Professional Women*. London, Croom Helm.

MacGuire, J. (1989). 'An approach to evaluating the introduction of primary nursing in an acute medical unit for the elderly – II Operationalising the Principles', *International Journal of Nursing Studies* **26**, 3, 253–60.

Mackay, L. (1989). *Nursing a Problem*. Milton Keynes, Open University Press.

McMahon, R. (1987). 'An analysis of power and collegial relations among nurses on wards implementing hierarchical and lateral management structures', unpublished MA dissertation, University of Warwick.

Maggs, C. (1983). *The Origins of General Nursing*. Beckenham, Croom Helm.

Malin, H. (1986). *Nurse Demand Methods – Wither Now?* DHSS Operational Research Service, London, DHSS.

Mann, M. (1983). *Macmillan Student Encyclopaedia of Sociology*. London, Macmillan.

Manthey, M. (1980). *The Practice of Primary Nursing*. Oxford, Blackwell.

Maslach, C. (1982). *Burnout: the Costs of Caring*. Englewood Cliffs, Prentice Hall.

Maynard, A. (1987). 'Health and economic research in the UK', in G. Teeling Smith (ed.) *Health Economics: Prospect for the Future*. 117–33, London, Croom Helm.

Medicines Act (1968). Chapter 67. London, HMSO.

Melia, K. (1987). *Learning and Working: the Occupational Socialisation of Nurses*. London, Tavistock.

Merry, P. (1990). 'Spirited defence of community health doctors', *British Medical Journal* **300**, 1591.

Metcalf, H. and Leighton, P. (1989). *The Underutilisation of Women in the Labour Market*. IMS Report No. 172, Brighton, Institute of Manpower Studies.

Ministry of Health (1920–39). *Annual Reports*. London, HMSO.

Ministry of Health MH55/1447 (1933). Admission of foreigners as probationer nurses to English hospitals. Letters from College of Nursing to Ministry of Health, 2 November, London, Public Record Office.

Ministry of Health (1944). *A National Health Service*. White Paper, Cmnd. 6502. London, HMSO.

Ministry of Health (1956). *Report of the Committee of Enquiry into the Cost of the National Health Service*. (Chairman, C.W. Guillebaud), Cmnd. 9663. London, HMSO.

Ministry of Health and Board of Education (1939). *Interim Report of the Interdepartmental Committee on Nursing Services*. (Chairman, The Earl of Athlone). London, HMSO.

Ministry of Health and Central Health Services Council (1954). *Report of the Committees on Internal Administration of Hospitals*. (Chairman, Alderman, A.F. Bradbeer), London, HMSO.

Ministry of Health, Ministry of Labour and National Service, Department of Health for Scotland (1943). *First Report of the Nurses' Salaries Committee.* (Chairman, Lord Rushcliffe), London, HMSO.

Ministry of Health, Ministry of Labour and National Service, Department of Health for Scotland (1947). *Report of the Working Party on the Recruitment and Training of Nurses.* London, HMSO.

Ministry of Health, Scottish Home and Health Department (1966). *Report of the Committee on Senior Nursing Staff Structure.* (Chairman, Brian Salmon), London, HMSO.

Ministry of Labour and National Service (1957). *Annual Report.* London, HMSO.

Mitchell, J. R. A. (1984). 'Is nursing any business of doctors? A simple guide to the "nursing process"', *British Medical Journal* **288**, 216–19.

National Audit Office (1985). 'National Health Service: Control of Nursing Manpower', *Report of the Comptroller and Auditor General.* London, HMSO.

National Audit Office (1990). *The NHS and Independent Hospitals.* London, HMSO.

National Economic Development Office (1988). *Young People and the Labour Market.* London, NEDO.

Nelson, J. (1976). 'Male domination ahead?', *Nursing Mirror* 15 April, **142**, 16, 69.

Nessling, B. and Boyle, S. (1990). 'Not so mobile a market', *Health Service Journal* 22 March, **100**.

Neter, J. and Wasserman, W. (1974). *Applied Linear Statistical Models.* Illinois, Irwin.

Nethercott, S. (1991). 'Up to date, but out of touch', *Nursing Times* 30 January, **87**, 5, 52–3.

Nottingham Journal and Express (1937). 'A revolt against hospital "tyranny"', 3 November.

Nurses, Midwives and Health Visitors Act (1979). London, HMSO.

Nursing Policy Studies Centre (1988). *Quadrennial Report 1985–1988.* NPSC, University of Warwick.

Nursing Standard (1988). 'Revised work boundaries urged', **2**, 32, 7.

Nursing Standard (1989). 'Role extension storm', **3**, 50, 5.

Nursing Times (1944). 'Nursing in our future health services: the professional conference', 9 December, 843–5.

O'Conner, J. (1988). 'Nurses respond to AMA proposal on new class of hospital workers', *Psychiatry News* **23**, 23.

Oakley, A. (1974). *Housewife.* Harmondsworth, Penguin.

Owen, P. and Glennister, H. (1990). *Nursing in Conflict.* London, Macmillan.

Pahl, R. (1984). *Divisions of Labour.* Oxford, Blackwell.

Parsons, T. (1951). *The Social System.* London, Routledge & Kegan Paul.

Pattie, A. and Gilleard, C. (1979). *Manual of the Clifton Assessment Procedures for the Elderly (CAPE).* Sevenoaks, Hodder & Stoughton.

Pearson, A. (1983). *The Clinical Nursing Unit.* London, Heinemann.

Pearson, A. (ed.) (1988). *Primary Nursing: Nursing in Burford and Oxford Nursing Development Units.* Beckenham, Croom Helm.

Pearson, A. *et al.* (1988) *Therapeutic Nursing: an Evaluation of an Experimental Nursing Unit in the British National Health Service.* Oxford, Burford and Oxford Nursing Development Units.

Pearson, A. *et al.* (1989). 'Determining quality in a unit where nursing is the primary intervention', *Journal of Advanced Nursing* **14**, 4, 269–73.

Pearson, M. (1987). 'Racism: the great divide', *Nursing Times* 17 June, **83**, 24, 24–6.

Pembrey, S. and Punton, S. (1990). 'The lessons of nursing beds', *Nursing Times* 4 April, **86**, 14, 44–5.

Pitkin, H. (1967). *The Concept of Representation*. University of California Press.

Porter, R. (1982). *English Society in the Eighteenth Century*. Harmondsworth, Penguin.

Porter, R. (1989). *Health for Sale: Quackery in England 1660–1850*. Manchester University Press.

Price Waterhouse (1987). *Report on the Costs, Benefits and Manpower Implications of Project 2000*. London, Price Waterhouse.

Rafferty, A. M. (1988). 'Nursing Policy and the Nationalisation of Nursing'. Paper presented to the Society for the Social History of Medicine conference on the National Health Service Institute for Historical Research, London.

Reed, S. (1988). 'A comparison of nurse-related behaviour, philosophy of care and job satisfaction in team and primary nursing', *Journal of Advanced Nursing* **13**, 3, 383–95.

Rein, M. (1983). *From Policy to Practice*. London, Macmillan.

Reverby, S. (1987). *Ordered to Care: the Dilemma of American Nursing, 1850–1945*. Cambridge University Press.

Robinson, J. (1979). 'Inter-disciplinary in-service education' (for health visitors and social workers), *Child Abuse and Neglect* **3**, 749–55.

Robinson, J. (1982). *An Evaluation of Health Visiting*. London, ENB/CETHV.

Robinson, J. (1989). 'Perinatal mortality – a report on a research study', *International Journal of Health Care Q A* **2**, 2, 13–19.

Robinson, J. (1990). 'Nursing in the future: a cause for concern?', in M. Jolley and P. Allan (eds) *Current Issues in Nursing*. London, Chapman & Hall.

Robinson, J. (1991). 'Power, politics and policy analysis in nursing', in A. Perry and M. Jolley (eds) *Nursing: a Knowledge Base for Practice*. London, Edward Arnold.

Robinson, J. and Elkan, R. (1989). *Research for Policy and Policy for Research: a Review of selected DHSS-funded Nurse Education Research 1975–1986*. Nursing Policy Studies 5, NPSC, University of Warwick.

Robinson, J. and Strong, P. (1987). *Professional Nursing Advice After Griffiths: An Interim Report*. Nursing Policy Studies 1, NPSC, University of Warwick.

Robinson, J. *et al.* (1989a). *Griffiths and the Nurses: A National Survey of CNAs*. Nursing Policy Studies 4, NPSC, University of Warwick.

Robinson, J. *et al.* (1989b). *The Role of the Support Worker in the Ward Health Care Team*. Nursing Policy Studies 6, NPSC, University of Warwick.

Robinson, K. and Rafferty, A. M. (1988). *The Nursing Workforce*. London, Polytechnic of the Southbank.

Rowbotham, S. (1973). *Women's Consciousness, Man's World*. London, Pelican.

Royal College of Nursing (1964). *A Reform of Nursing Education*. (Chairman, Sir Harry Platt), First Report of a Special Committee on Nurse Education, London, RCN.

Royal College of Nursing and British Medical Association (1978). *The Duties and Position of the Nurse*. Revised edition, London, RCN and BMA.

Salaman, G. (1979). *Work Organizations: Resistance and Control*. Harlow, Longman.

Salvage, J. (1985). *The Politics of Nursing*. London, Heinemann Nursing.

Salvage, J. (1988). 'Professionalisation – or struggle for survival? A consideration of current proposals for the reform of nursing in the UK', *Journal of Advanced Nursing* **13**, 4, 515–19.

Salvage, J. (1989). 'Setback for nursing', *Nursing Times* 15 March, **85**, 11, 19.

Salvage, J. (1990a). 'The theory and practice of the "New Nursing"', *Nursing Times* Occasional Paper, 24 January, **86**, 4, 42–5.
Salvage, J. (1990b). 'Treating the malaise in time', *Health Services Journal* **100**, 84–5.
Scottish Office (1990). *Scottish Abstract of Statistics 1989*. Edinburgh, HMSO.
Sear, H. J. and Williams, S. (forthcoming). 'Managerial implications of primary nursing', in E. Tutton and S. Ersser (eds) *Primary Nursing in Perspective*. London, Scutari.
Sharpe, S. (1984). *Double Identity: the Lives of Working Mothers*. Harmondsworth, Pelican.
Sheaff, R. (1991). *Marketing for Health Services*. Milton Keynes, Open University Press.
Shipp, P. (1989). *Health Personnel Projections: The Methods and Their Uses*. Geneva, World Health Organization.
Shuttleworth, A. (1988). 'Job sharing can take the strain out of recruitment', *The Professional Nurse* November, **4**, 2, 68–70.
Silverman, D. (1970). *The Theory of Organisations*. London, Heinemann.
Sixsmith, A. *et al.* (1990). *District Experimental Care Schemes for the Elderly Mentally Ill, a Report to the Department of Health*. Liverpool, Institute for Human Ageing.
Skinner, D. V. (1985). 'Cardiopulmonary resuscitation skills of pre-registration house officers', *British Medical Journal* **290**, 1549–50.
Smail, R. and Gray, A. M. (1982). *Nurses' Pay in the NHS*. Health Economics Unit, University of Aberdeen.
Smith, P. (1988). 'Quality of nursing and the ward as a learning environment for student nurses: a multimethod approach', unpublished PhD thesis, University of London.
Smith, P. (1991). 'The nursing process: raising the profile of emotional care in nurse training', *Journal of Advanced Nursing* **16**, 1, 74–81.
Smith, P. and Redfern, S. (1989). 'The quality of care and students' educational experience in hospital wards', in J. Wilson-Barnett and S. Robinson (eds) *Directions in Nursing Research*. London, Scutari Press.
Stacey, M. (1988). *The Sociology of Health and Healing*. London, Unwin Hyman.
Stein, L. I. (1967). 'The doctor–nurse game', *Archive of General Psychiatry* **16**, 699–703.
Stein, L. I. *et al.* (1990). 'The doctor–nurse game revisited', *New England Journal of Medicine* **322**, 546–9.
Stoddard, S. (1979). *The Hospice Movement*. London, Cape.
Strauss, A. *et al.* (1985). *Social Organization of Medical Work*. University of Chicago Press.
Strong, P. and Robinson, J. (1988). *New Model Management: Griffiths and the NHS*. Nursing Policy Studies 3, NPSC, University of Warwick.
Strong, P. and Robinson, J. (1990). *The NHS Under New Management*. Milton Keynes, Open University Press.
Thompson, P. (1983). *The Nature of Work*. London, Macmillan.
The Times (1988). 'Patients "put at risk" by long hours', 27 December, 3.
Torkington, P. (1987). 'Sorry, wrong colour', *Nursing Times* 17 June, **83**, 24, 27–8.
Trades Union Congress (1937). *Report of Proceedings of 69th Annual Trade Union Conference*. London, TUC.
Turner, B. (1987). *Medical Power and Social Knowledge*. London, Sage.
Turnock, C. (1991). 'Communicating with patients in ICU', *Nursing Standard* **5**, 15/16, 38–40.
Tutton, L. (1986). 'What is primary nursing?', *Professional Nurse* November, **2**, 2, 39–40.
UKCC (1986a). *Project 2000: A New Preparation for Practice*. London, UKCC.

UKCC (1986b). *Administration of Medicines*. London, UKCC.

UKCC (1987). *Project 2000: The Final Proposals*. London, UKCC.

Ungerson, C. (1983). 'Women and caring: skills, tasks and taboos', in E. Gamarnikow, D. Morgan and J. Purvis (eds) *The Public and the Private*. London, Heinemann.

Ungerson, C. (1987). *Policy is Personal*. London, Tavistock.

Upton, P. (1989). 'House Officers' workload – little change in 20 years', *Health Bulletin* **47**, 179–81.

Vachon, M. (1987). *Occupational Stress in the Care of the Critically Ill, the Dying and the Bereaved*. New York, Hemisphere.

Waite, R. (forthcoming). *Role Flexibility and Skill Mix*. Brighton, Institute of Manpower Studies.

Waite, R. and Pike, G. (1989). *School Leaver Decline and Effective Local Solutions*. IMS Report No. 178, Brighton, Institute of Manpower Studies.

Waite, R. *et al.* (1989). *Nurses In and Out of Work*. IMS Report No. 170, Brighton, Institute of Manpower Studies.

Waite, R. *et al.* (1990). *The Career and Patterns of Scotland's Qualified Nurses*. Scottish Home and Health Department/IMS.

Walby, S. (1987). *Flexibility and the Changing Division of Labour*. Lancaster Regionalism Group Working Paper 36, University of Lancaster.

Webb, C. (1985). *Sexuality, Nursing and Health*. Chichester, Wiley.

Webster, C. (1985). 'Nursing and the crisis of the early National Health Service', *Bulletin in the History of Nursing* **Group** 7, 4–12.

Webster, C. (1988). *Problems of Health Care: The British National Health Service Before 1957*. London, HMSO.

Welsh Office (1987). *Second Report of the All Wales Nurse Manpower Planning Committee*. Cardiff, Welsh Office.

Welsh Office (1990). *Health and Personal Social Services for Wales*, No. 16. Cardiff, Welsh Office.

White, R. (1985). *Political Issues in Nursing: Past, Present and Future*, Vol. 1. Chichester, Wiley.

White, R. (1986a). *Political Issues in Nursing: Past, Present and Future*, Vol. 2. Chichester, Wiley.

White, R. (1986b). *The Effects of the NHS on the Nursing Profession 1948–1961*. King's Fund Historical Series, Oxford University Press.

White, R. (1988). *Political Issues in Nursing: Past, Present and Future*. Vol. 3. Chichester, Wiley.

Williams, K. (1974). 'Ideologies of nursing: their meanings and implications', *Nursing Times* Occasional Paper, 8 August.

Williams, K. (1980). 'From Sarah Gamp to Florence Nightingale: a critical study of hospital nursing systems from 1840 to 1897' in C. Davies (ed.) *Rewriting Nursing History*. London, Croom Helm.

Wilkes, E. (1986). 'Introduction', *Terminal Care*. Update Postgraduate Centre Series, Guildford, Update-Siebert.

Wilkin, D. and Jolley, D. (1979). *Behavioural Problems Among Old People in Geriatric Wards, Psychogeriatric Wards and Residential Homes 1976–1978*. Research Report 1, Manchester University Hospital of South Manchester.

Wilson-Barnett, J. (1988). 'Nursing values: exploring the clichés', *Journal of Advanced Nursing* **13**, 6, 790–6.

Woodham-Smith, C. (1950). *Florence Nightingale 1820–1910.* London, Constable.

Wouters, C. (1990). 'Changing regimes of power and emotions at the end of life: The Netherlands 1930–1990', unpublished paper, Netherlands, Department of General Social Sciences, University of Utrecht.

Wright, S. (1986). *Building and Using a Model for Nursing.* London, Edward Arnold.

Yett, D. (1975). *An Economic Analysis of the Nursing Shortage.* Lexington, Mass., Lexington Books.

Young, A. (1976). 'Some implications of medical beliefs and practices for social anthropology', *American Anthropologist* 78, 1, 5–24.

Index